MASTER THE DAY

MASTER THE

DAY

Eat, Move and Live Better With
The Power of Daily Habits

ALEXANDER HEYNE

To all the people who struggle every day to figure out how to get from where they are, to where they want to be.

CONTENTS

Prologue

1

2

3

4

5

10

11

12

13

14

Epilogue

What Others Are Saying About Master the Day

"Hi Alex, if you remember me my name is Boris and I am from Indonesia and I sent you an email about a year ago. I just wanted to say thanks for all the advice you shared on your website because after implementing them I went from 103kg (227 pounds) in May 2014 to 86kg (190 pounds) as of December 2014. One thing that I learned from all this is that diet is not a goal but is a lifelong process that includes changing one's mindset and lifestyle."

- BORIS, S. - INDONESIA.

"Hi Alex,

I follow your stuff and I have to say... it's awesome. You go into much more depth than many other diet books or programs by discussing the psychology of losing weight. I think that the mind is 90 percent of the battle, because the body will respond to any change a person makes.

For me the hardest part is getting started and staying motivated. Before watching your videos, I would try to stay perfect, completely overhauling everything in my diet for X amount of days, but when I had one bad day and ate junk food, I felt like I just lost all my progress, so I would give up for period of time, until I decided that I want to get healthy again. It is a horrible cycle and one that I want to break.

So thank you for the actionable advice."

- SANDRA, M. - LONDON

"Hi Alex,

I wanted to let you know, that, before I found [this approach], I was burdened with the thought of weight loss every day. I had put on a few kilos last year & whatever I tried I could not lose it. It was always on my mind & was affecting my life. After reading your advice I don't even worry about my weight any more and have lost a couple of kilos! I can also fit into a pair of jeans that were too tight last year -- I am very happy with the lifestyle I have now, thanks to you."

- Kathy, S. - UK

"I've been slowly integrating your teachings into my eating and have, for the first time in a long time, seen some results on the scale. I weighed in this morning… in the last 1.5 to 2 weeks… I have lots about 5-6 pounds. But also, I was thinking I lost a whole lot more because of how I feel. I feel lighter… my stomach feels flatter… I used to go down the stairs kind of on leg at a time holding onto the rail. This morning… right down… one foot after the other. Very encouraging."

- Mark, A. – Kentucky, USA.

"Hi Alex – I've started following your advice each day and I've lost 6 pounds in 6 days – I'm pretty sure all these things have had a huge impact already hence the weight loss without any dieting or exercise at all. Once again, tonnes of thank you's for your hard work and advice."

- Nel, R. Australia.

The Elephant In the Room: What Nobody Wants to Tell You About Looking & Feeling Incredible

What you're about to learn are the *facts* I discovered after interviewing and studying dozens of people that lost 100+ pounds naturally, without diet fads, and kept it off years later. These principles transform much more than just a person's health, and they aren't just abstract ideas I made up after an "aha" moment in the shower one day. They're also based on hundreds of my own students and clients – and the key traits behind which ones succeed or fail in the long run. These two principles don't care if you started rich or poor; they don't care if you're miserable or happy, fat or skinny.

They don't care how much education you had or how little education you had. They don't care if you're French or American, Chinese or African, Mexican or Filipino. And most of all, these keys are just as effective if you're twenty-two or sixty, a man or a woman, a busy CEO or have all the time in the world.

When I introduce you to them, you'll see for yourself just how powerful they can be as tools to transform your health and your life forever.

***

June 15, 1954.

Two beautiful twins are born into the world. Their names are Billy and Michelle. They're both born into the same social class, middle class. They are both raised by great parents in a loving and supportive household. They both go to the same school, and hang out with the same friends. They eat the same potluck dinner every night, and play the same sports. They take the same vacations, and even read the same books. They're both into personal development so they read at least one great book per month. They both get married and go on to have kids, and create warm, loving families that celebrate the holidays together. They both read the same magazines, watch the same TV shows, and they even go to many of the same events as adults.

But here's where they differ: Despite all their similarities, over the decades, Michelle has maintained her slim 135-pound physique with very little variation over the years. She enjoys incredible health – she's bursting with energy that allows her to juggle her career and a family and still maintain her sanity. She sleeps soundly at night, with the worries of her own life and the world not keeping her up. She's pretty much never had a muffin top – and even now, at 48, even though she's gained a tiny bit of weight she still looks years younger than she really is.

She also has almost half a million dollars saved, everyone describes her as "so happy she could be on Prozac," and she seems to have it all.

Her brother Billy, however, is a different story altogether. Even though Billy and Michelle were both at a healthy weight in their twenties (when it's easy), Billy is now fifty pounds overweight, with high blood pressure, pre-diabetes, sleep apnea, a spastic colon, no sex drive, and zero energy. In fact, he doesn't even remember what being healthy felt like – since all he deals with every day is constant, impenetrable fatigue and brain fog that hits him the second he wakes up.

Despite earning a strong six-figure income for the last decade, he is over $50,000 in debt, with virtually no savings. And to top it off, he's known as the scrooge of his town, always complaining about the things going wrong for him, about how hard *he* works and how little *he* gets in return.

What gives? How could two people with a similar IQ and upbringing, with similar interests, education and parenting styles end up so different? How did Michelle's life appear to get better with age – with incredible levels of health and vitality, physical wealth, happiness and an amazing family? It wasn't just her net worth or health that got better. It was her *life* net worth. And how could Billy seem like a pawn thrown around in the wind by an angry deity? What is he missing that she possesses?

In this book, I am going to introduce you to the key that Michelle possessed.

What I Learned Interviewing 20+ People That Lost Over 100 Pounds And Kept it Off Years Later (Without Calorie Counting or Fad Diets)

There's a big 'secret' that the healthiest, happiest people on the planet get that most of us don't. And I'm not talking about these silly fitness models spamming your social media newsfeed saying, *"If you aren't pushing until you die, you're weak!"* I'm talking about just average people like you and me - average people that transformed their health and their life. It might surprise you that their health and weight loss had little to do with forcing themselves to eat less, move more, or any of the typical diet advice you get from the magazine tabloids at the grocery store. Not a single one of these people counted calories.

In fact, it was just the opposite. And it was the result of only two principles. These two principles I noticed over and over as I interviewed dozens of case studies before finally putting the pieces together myself.

***

In 2013, on a beautiful August day, I strolled into my local bookstore because I had a burning question nagging me. *"Why is it, despite the fact that we have twenty-five new "shred diet" books by mysterious M.D.s this year, people are getting bigger and sicker than ever, and aren't any more successful at looking and feeling a lot better?"* It blew my mind that virtually everyone on the planet had access to all of the information since the dawn of humanity, yet we were apparently no closer to the health and physical appearance that we so often craved. In other words, in a world where virtually *everyone* has access to all the information *ever* released on the planet, why do only a couple percent succeed at actually having the pain-free, vital, strong, slim body they want?

Think about it. If we all have access to the world's store of information, why aren't we all millionaires, happy, slim, and content? All the information is there. That's when I realized that information meant very little. The diet (the information) we chose usually had very little (or limited) impact on the bottom line: the body and health we wanted. That's when I realized why I had a stack of books on happiness ten feet tall, yet day-to-day I complained about being mildly unhappy.

That was the day I realized that many of us have read finance books or have at one point wondered how to make more money, but most of us aren't where we want to be financially.

Why aren't they telling us this? I sat down for a second and just stared at the health and wellness rack in the bookstore. "What if the diet had nothing to do with it? What if 'dieting' really had little to do with the diet, and instead had more to do with *life*?" All of these gurus were giving the same advice: what to actually do, but no one was saying *how* to actually do it. Pieces began to connect. How *do* the successful few do it?

I was hooked. I wanted to figure out this key for myself: so I set out upon a mission. I sought out, interviewed, studied and analyzed dozens of people (20+) that lost 100+ pounds naturally, kept it off years later, didn't go on a fad diet or count calories, and did it just by changing certain key habits. I got on the phone with each of these people, recorded the calls, and played the 30+ hours of calls back a dozen times each. As a certified personal trainer, an undergraduate biology major from a top university, and a guy that has been in the gym for almost a decade, I wasn't coming in to this blind. I had a rough idea of what I *thought* they were going to say.

I asked them similar things originally. At first, I had the same questions you might have. "What were you eating? How much? How often? How did you control portions? What kind of exercises were you doing? How many times a week? How did you deal with cravings, sweets, and negative friends?" Strangely enough, these conversations almost never came up when I asked them. I was puzzled. If they didn't solely attribute the diet (what they ate, or how much), or the exercise plan to their insane results… what were they doing? What was *their secret?* As I got through interview #10 I began noticing some interesting trends. What I picked up on in one story, I would then go playback in another interview and see if it was present there too.

Here's what I discovered: I learned that they *all* engaged in the same few habits. I learned that *some* of them had a few unique habits. And I learned that *none* of them embodied certain key habits you'd think they would (like calorie counting). But I noticed one key trend surrounding all of their success stories. It's the one big key I talked about earlier. And that one principle (the *only* principle they all had in common), was that they understood that sustainable health and weight loss came down to two things, and two things only:

Here's what that key was - it was a combination of understanding the person's inner psychology (what I call *"The Narrative"* with a capital "T"), and their understanding of tiny habits. From now on, when I refer to *The Key*, you'll know that it means *The Inner Narrative (Your Psychology) + Tiny Daily Habits.* Interestingly enough, there's no mention of a diet anywhere in there. There's no mention of eating less or moving more. Here's why: At the end of the day, what's less important is what diet we're on as long as we're eating real food.

Several years ago, a Yale professor was chartered to analyze many of the major diet trends and see which one was most effective. What he and his team found was that it didn't matter if the person went low fat, low carb, or low something else. What mattered was that they were *carb* and *fat selective* – meaning, they just chose the right healthy ones, rather than removing them.[1]

They didn't remove fat; they just ate the fats found in proper meats as well as foods like avocado and nuts (rather than trans fats). They didn't remove carbs; they just ate the proper low GI carbs, like brown rice, instead of white bread. Another study tried to figure out something similar: which diet is most actually most effective at weight loss long term? The study done in the Journal of the American Medical Association found the following after comparing a few popular diets: the major thing predicting your levels of health and weight loss is your ability to adhere to whatever plan you have set forth – more than the diet itself.[2]

Crazy, huh? It was almost like the information they had – the diet – had little effect on their success. It was just whether the person *did* what they said they would. And I hate to break it to you – but that one's an inner game. That one's on us. This book will show you how: and it will give you that key. *The Key.*

Chapter Recap: "The Big Secret"

☐ The two "success principles" discovered after interviewing dozens of people that lost 100+ pounds and kept it off years later (improving more than just weight) were:

☐ 1. **An understanding of** *The Narrative* – that story we keep telling ourselves – and how it causes us to make the same mistakes over and over, or how it discourages us constantly. There was a big emphasis on paying attention to the narrative, and re-writing it.

☐ 2. **An emphasis on changing behavior, and habits, not weight loss tips, tricks, diets or fads.** The case studies I interviewed emphasized going back to the true origin: our behavior, rather than the diet. If something didn't work, what habits or behaviors led us down that road?

A Sneak Peek of What's In This Book And How You Can Use it to Transform Your Life

This book is organized into two main parts. The first half is all about what's been holding us back from being the huge success we want to be (and we can be) from a health and weight loss perspective. This part of the book is mostly about how (and why) we often fail to reach our health, weight loss, and life goals, and what to do about it.

The second phase of the book is all about the crunchy techniques, tactics, and daily habits you can apply beginning today to stick to healthy habits, get your dream body, and finally *get your life back* and no longer wonder "how did I even get here?" In chapter one, we're going to talk about getting from where you are to where you want to be. I'm going to introduce you to my "it's just not about eating less and moving more" philosophy, and then show you the power of just getting 1% better each day.

From there we'll jump right into what I call *The Horsemen*. The Horsemen part of the book is all about the repetitive negative habits holding us back from our dreams of better health (that we may not even realize have been sabotaging us). Consider these the horsemen of the health apocalypse. If you've ever failed repeatedly to reach your goals, have yo-yo dieted for decades, and find yourself always starting back at square one and repeating the same goals over and over, this part of the book will be invaluable. We all fall prey to these at one point or another in our lives, but maybe this will "re-awaken" the awareness of it. A big part of this chapter will be dispelling one huge, pervasive myth: The willpower and discipline myth.

After this first part of the book, we'll jump into part two. The second part is all about the solution: why we fail, and what to do about it. Like I said, I promised you a diet-free way to create habits that help you create success *that's sustainable and permanent*. In part two, I'll walk you through several daily habits that have either been adapted directly from my interviews with these 100+ pound weight loss success stories, or have been some of the most important principles in my most successful students and clients. This is also where I introduce you to the key philosophy in this book and how to apply it: *"The Narrative"* + Little Daily Habits. From there, I give you the *Master the Day: Million Dollar Daily Ritual* to stay focused and motivated, and show you how to stay consistent on the long road ahead, when life will inevitably try to intervene with your master plan.

It's going to be an exciting journey, so go ahead, jump in and get started.

Why This Is Probably The Only Diet Book Without a Diet and Workout Plan

You might be surprised. Nowhere in this book am I giving you a meal plan, diet guide, workouts, or tips and tactics based on your body type. Actually, to be specific, there's only *one* page where I suggest what to eat (at the very end). Why? It's simple: Chances are, you already know what you need to eat, what exercises to do, what tiny habits to ingrain, but you just aren't doing them.

The reason we fail is not just because we are eating the wrong foods or doing the wrong exercises. The reason we fail is because we keep changing the diet, the guru, the scheme, the strategy, without changing *ourselves as individuals*. Let me repeat that. The reason we fail to be healthy isn't because of the food and exercise, the diet plan or the lack of the diet plan (even though you obviously need those).

We fail because we keep changing *what* we do, without changing *who we are.* Think about it. When a relationship is going sour in our life, we can get all these core tactics: be more romantic, pay attention to our partner's needs, blah blah blah. But at the end of the day, if our bad temper is the reason for arguments, there is no tip or trick on the planet that can fix the relationship. We need to fix the temper. If we're insanely insecure, there isn't a guru on the planet that could fix the relationship unless we change that aspect of our self. Band-Aids just won't work.

Well the same is true of health. If we're struggling to "stick" with a diet plan or regime, it really has little to do with the diet (even though it may be *insanely* restrictive, no fun, or not based on science). We might procrastinate and say, "Ehh I'll get around to it soon. I'll do phase two in a few weeks." Sometimes we have this repetitive story going on that says, "I always fail, so why bother trying yet again? I might as well just enjoy the stuff I like." Or we might get home late from work and say, "I'll just get some takeout, it's late and I'm exhausted." Or it's time to go for our walk and that resistance crops up telling us, "Just snooze for ten more minutes." Sometimes it's just a boring, tiring, stressful or hormonal day and we *really need* that treat to pep us up.

Eventually, as the typical lifecycle of the dieter goes, we repeat diet plan after diet plan without ever getting any closer to where we want to be. It's all because we keep changing *what* we're doing, the tips, tactics, techniques, without changing *who we are*. We never really address the underlying cause. In other words, we can change the guru, the plan, the diet, the book, the strategy, or the workout a hundred times. But nothing changes for good unless our *behavior* changes for good. If we don't change, nothing changes – no matter how many times we introduce a new game plan. What we do every single day, whether consciously or unconsciously, creates the life we have today. We bounce from shiny object to shiny object, guru to guru, without every addressing the fundamental underlying cause of failure and success: us.

It's not *what* we do, but *whether or not we do it* (and why) that prevents us from getting to where we want to be. And here's a truth most people won't tell you: It's largely a psychological game, dictated by the thoughts, fears, and beliefs in our head. What's more, the *story* you tell yourself about why your health is the way it is, is infinitely more powerful than the truth.

What I'm hoping this book will awaken in you is simple: the awareness that succeeding at getting healthy, and getting your dream body (for life), is an inside game. It always was. And it isn't until we change who we fundamentally are as a person - our habits, beliefs, mindset, and behaviors – can we finally access the success we want.

CHAPTER 1

Getting From Where You Are To Where You Want to Be - The Power of 1% Better

"The boy didn't know what a person's "destiny" was. It's what you have always wanted to accomplish. Everyone, when they are young, knows what their destiny is. At that point in their lives, everything is clear and everything is possible. They are not afraid to dream, and to yearn for everything they would like to see happen to them in their lives. But, as time passes, a mysterious force begins to convince them that it will be impossible for them to realize their destiny."

– The Alchemist

You're here reading this for a reason. First of all, you're a human being. You have goals, but achieving them is another story entirely. Sometimes you feel like a continual failure, like you were dreaming too big and "now it's time to play it safe and be realistic." You have dreams, but for some reason they seem out of reach – more like a fantasy than an inevitable reality you are working towards.

You want more from life – more everything. Better health, more fulfilling relationships, different vacations (or maybe just a vacation), a better job, a higher salary, more meaning and more purpose. But you want one thing in particular if you're reading this: no matter what you say to yourself or your friends, what you really want deep down is to be proud of who you are. You want to look incredible, and feel like a million bucks.

You want to take thirty seconds when you get out of shower and catch a sneak peek of yourself and go, *"Damn, I look good!"* You want that childlike feeling of sleeping like a baby again – waking up with crazy energy, loads of energy that leaves you feeling like you can conquer the world each day. You want freedom from food; you want to be able to eat the right foods, when you want, without cravings, without feeling like food controls your entire life.

You're tired of dealing with sketchy health sites that contradict everything from the next site. You're hardly thrilled about removing carbs and other food groups and calling that a "sustainable" diet plan. You're a busy professional, parent, or stressed out mom juggling multiple lives: professional, personal, health, and more. So finding the *time* to do all these things is your primary consideration.

You're tired of the "rah rah" *fitspiration* BS telling you to work harder until you die, showing disgustingly fit people that are hardly inspiring – they just inspire resentment. You're tired of dealing with restrictive advice that promises to "change your life" and then gives you a list of 4,567 foods you can't eat – making you wonder what you actually *can* eat. Since when did a "big list of things I can't eat and a meal plan" ever work for anyone?

You want something that gives you the tools to succeed *in the long run* and actually *maintain* your progress for life. You want a strategy unique to you and your circumstances, because how could a 45-year-old busy mother get the same health regime that a 22-year-old single man got? And most of all, you want something *realistic* that doesn't eliminate all the fun of life, eating, and going out with your friends. You want something real, and you want something sustainable. Chances are, you're also kind of uncertain how you got where you are today. It sort of seems like one day you just woke up in someone else's body, (and maybe someone else's life) – one day you woke up and realized, *"Wow, how did I get to this point? How did it get this bad?"* Maybe you're a bit heavier than you realized – twenty or thirty pounds over your natural body weight. Maybe health problems have been cropping up like acid reflux, some GI issues, back pain, massive fatigue and lack of energy.

Or maybe your health is just one symptom of a larger problem in your life: *"How on earth did I get here?"* It almost all feels like a bad dream - like you woke up in someone else's life. "I wake up, take a shower, make breakfast, sit in traffic, go to the 9-5 job, come home, watch TV, rinse and repeat. And on and on my life goes like this. Every day it's the same thing, Groundhog Day repeated over and over again. What happened to that incredible, inspirational life I envisioned when I was young? *What happened to me?"*

***

> *"Compound interest is the eighth wonder of the world. He who understands it, earns it ... he who doesn't ... pays it."*
>
> - ALBERT EINSTEIN

It's known as life's best-kept secret. You've heard of the power of compound interest, I'm sure. You've heard about all this stuff about "saving early" because it'll make you rich later. But what almost no one talks about is *compound habit interest*. We know that saving a bit of money each day creates big rewards that only a small percentage of the planet enjoys.

But what about the *tiny daily habits* that produce these huge rewards? Habits so small that they don't even seem worthwhile. Habits that seem almost entirely unrelated to getting healthier or losing some weight. Habits that, from the outside, don't seem to do anything, but compounded produce Olympians, Best-selling authors, or plain old average men and women with incredible health and fulfilling lives. Let's take one of those tiny habits many of us *know* we should be doing, but often aren't doing, and take a look at what it looks like thirty years down the road. Let's say you plop down $1,000 of your savings into an account or an investment. And let's say you add a very conservative $100 a month into this savings account that is compounding at 5% annually.

Here's what that would look like after ten years:

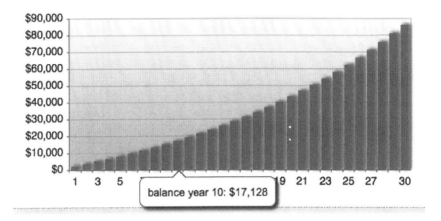

balance year 10: $17,128

After twenty years:

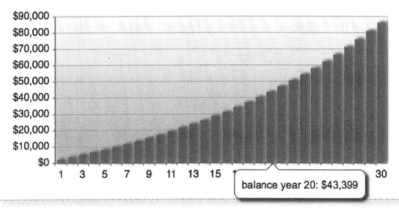

balance year 20: $43,399

After thirty years:

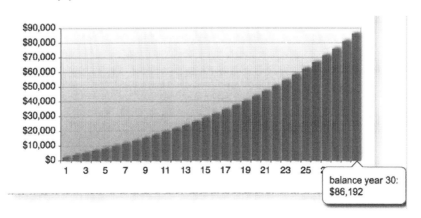

balance year 30: $86,192

So after thirty years, even though you only invested $37,000 of your own money, you almost tripled it at around $86,192 – because you *consistently added to the pot*. You've likely heard this scenario before, and your parents have probably drilled it into you. Yet after I interviewed the success stories I mentioned earlier in the book, I became curious: what about compound *habit* interest? What happens when you pick one easy, five-minute habit, and you do it daily for thirty years? Or what about just for a year? What does your life look like?

That's what I want you to consider as you read through this book.

Being healthy, happy, and feeling incredible doesn't take massive time, willpower or discipline. It just takes *compound habit interest*, a few little things you do each day without fail, consistently, over time. Success doesn't lie on the other side of massive willpower or discipline. It just relies on tiny daily habits, and the decisions we make every single moment.

Sorry, It's Not (Just) About Eating Less and Moving More

Weight loss is not just about eating less and moving more, *it's about life*. Here's what I mean: Consider the busy mom who has two full-time gigs. Janey is a super busy power mom with two full-time jobs: being a marketing director for a local nonprofit as well as being a full-time mom. The mornings are spent rushed and stressed – as always – yelling at her kids to get them out of bed (they're almost teenagers now), making them breakfast, and ushering them out the door. She grabs a piece of toast with butter and her morning coffee at home, but if she's really rushed she'll grab a coffee and whatever goodies are behind the counter at the local coffee shop or at the office.

As a high up role at her current job, she's under tons of stress to meet deadlines, and that only gets worse as she comes back home where she has "dinner" deadlines and "homework" deadlines. By the end of the night, she's so exhausted that all she wants is a piece of chocolate and a glass or two of wine. Prepare for tomorrow? *"You've got to be kidding me."* Today just ended and it's 9:30 pm.

Would a diet help her?

Think about it. Is changing what she ate each day going to help this extreme workload, which is honestly the origin of her poor eating habits? Or is it the stressed out, overbooked lifestyle what needs changing in order for her to be successful and where she wants to be with her health? Later in this book you're going to hear about one of my students, Mike, who was a stressed out professional working twelve hours a day at a new job to prove his worth to his new boss. Mike would get up at eight, leave the house at nine, and wouldn't get back home until twelve hours later – around nine PM. The collective stress of working twelve, crushing, pressured hours per day left him fried, and by the time he got home he was burnt to a crisp: some quick Chinese takeout and a few bottles of beer were required.

Required.

He couldn't function without his daily de-stress ritual, otherwise he found himself getting snappy at his wife which made him feel guilty. What was he supposed to do? The food just made him feel better. Can a diet help him? *Would* a diet help him? Was the diet the origin of Mike's health problems and recent weight gain, or was it his overworked lifestyle? Was it the food or the lifestyle that caused this de-railed life?

Here's one more example. Michelle is a 27-year-old professional who works as an account manager for a corporate company in New York City. Ah, *corporate* life. To be honest, she dreads it. She dreads the entire white picket fence life, waking up at the same time every day, sitting in the same old rush hour traffic, talking to the same people, working on the same projects, repeating life every day like groundhog day. It's gotten to the point where it's starting to really sap her energy on a daily basis. She knows she needs to quit because her soul is being sucked dry and her creative juices are… wait, what creative juices? But she's really afraid, and she worked so hard to get there and get a stable job like her parents never had.

Interestingly enough, any time she finds herself working on a particular project at work around 3:15 pm, she walks over to the cafeteria, grabs a cookie and a soda, and then walks around for a few minutes before getting back to work. It happens daily like clockwork. And after she gets home and can decompress to some reality TV, she pours herself a glass of wine or two and sometimes a bowl of ice cream, and melts into the sofa. *"It's the only three hours of my life I actually enjoy,"* she laments. How does changing Michelle's diet help her? Is it *really* the origin of her recent fifteen-pound weight gain?

Would a diet help her?

Is changing Michelle's diet the magical solution to her problems? Is that really going to reverse her recent weight gain, or does she just need to change her job? This is one of those big "secrets" or rather *facts* that no one wants to know about. Ninety-day workout plans can't save us. The Paleo diet can't save us. Low carb, low fat, and low fun can't save us. In fact, *this may sound* strange, but it was never about the diet. It's about us.

It's only once we change the inner story in our head, and we understand the systems, habits and life circumstances leading us down the road we're on now will we finally make it happen in our life. Ultimately, our weight and our health is just a reflection of one thing: our behavior, and our behavior is dictated by our daily choices, which become habits. Incredible health doesn't have to be hard or time consuming, it just means that we have to wake up, pay attention, and change those tiny decisions we make each day.

The Philosopher's Stone, Parisian Villas, And Living The *Really* Good Life

How did we get here, anyway? Think about it for just a moment. *How did I get here?* How did it ever get this bad? How did I get to this point? Ideally think about your health for a moment, but you can ponder any aspect of your life. If your relationship isn't satisfactory, how did it get this way? It wasn't always this way, was it? If you aren't that happy, how did you become this way? At one point or another in your life, every day was incredible, wasn't it?

Even if you have to think all the way back to childhood, at some point, life was awesome. And now, think about your health.

Who is that person in the mirror?
Where did they come from?
How did they get here inside my skin?

How on earth did it get to this point? "On some level I knew it was happening... but that didn't stop it from happening," we often say. What happened? Sometimes when we wake up with the feeling that we're in someone else's life, it's important to pause for a second and think: what series of events got me here? Usually, three things happened that lead to the classic "how did I get here?" moment.

First – we made certain choices, with or without realizing it. When you think about it, every larger aspect of our life is just an accumulation of thousands of tiny choices we made, usually over years. Getting a little bit of a muffin top or beer belly? Usually we made the decision to grab that muffin at the coffee shop in the morning or go out with the guys for beer after work. Do that a couple times a week (or once a week), and there's a new person in your body after a few years. Sometimes, choices can be sneaky. More often than not, our choices are unconscious. One of my clients once called this the "autopilot lifestyle" which I think sums it up pretty nicely. Sometimes drinking six cups of coffee is *just what you do* at your job if you're a busy professional or working in a startup. Sometimes getting that little cookie in the afternoon is *just part of your afternoon routine*. Sometimes snapping at your spouse when she reminds you about something you didn't do *is just the way your routine goes*. Nonetheless, more than anything, our choices (whether conscious or not) are the origin of who and what we are today.

Second – our choices became certain habits. The second thing that I'm going to focus on extensively here is the power of habits. We all know that we make dozens (or hundreds) of choices throughout the day that impact our lives. But what we may not realize is that these choices, when made frequent enough, solidify into habits and hardwire pathways into the brain.

The decision to smoke a cigarette when we're stressed or bored originally became a choice – which then became a habit (on many levels). The same decision to go to food for relief when we're depressed or sad can become a choice enough times that this too becomes an emotional eating habit. The decision to stay up and do an extra hour of work after our kids are in bed, scrolling through our phone and computer email, and then being unable to sleep, starts as a choice then becomes a habit. And much like the coffee drinker, at some point we just consider it "the way things have always been."

The funny thing is this: we actually act surprised when the meltdown occurs. In fact, the meltdown was building the entire time, just so slow that we couldn't notice it – like aging. We'll talk more on this later.

Third, we settled into the autopilot lifestyle (AL) and forgot to live deliberately. Mostly, this whole "how did I get here" thing boils down to one big thing: not living life deliberately. For many us, mediocre (or poor) health is just a reflection of the state of our lives.

Job? Eh. Relationship? Eh. Health? Eh. *Life?* Eh. Let's be honest: it's really easy for us to get caught up in the autopilot life. Sometimes it feels like any (and all) of the years after college or school were a whirlwind. We finished school, eager to conquer the world with our big dreams and passions, and then got sucked into the grind of getting a job. After sticking with the job and getting secure, we promised ourselves we'd travel, but most of us fell in love and got married: and now it's family time. Soon enough, shifting between the job and the family time, there wasn't much time left to do anything else. At the end of the long day juggling both, it's hard to resist the temptation of plopping down on the couch to resist the oncoming coma of fatigue. After working nine or ten hours, then coming home to a partner that needs supporting and kids that need disciplining and attention, who has time for anything else?

It happens to the best of us. Unfortunately, all too often, one day we wake up and look in the mirror and go: "Whoa. That's me? *But how…?*" And when we see our body (and think about how we feel), we realize that *life*, and not just our health, has followed suit. The autopilot life caught up with us. It might surprise you if I told you that most of these case studies that went on to have impressive physical transformations also had *impressive life transformations*. When they decided *"no more autopilot lifestyle,"* they started living deliberately. Like I said, this book is about way more than just weight loss or health. It's about the most precious thing we all have – life.

The remedy, the antidote, is deliberate living. It's waking up and thinking, "What do I really want from life? How do I *actually* want to look and feel every single day?" It's taking the time to be *deliberate* in thought and action about what you want, and how you can get there. It's time to sit down for a minute and think: what's the coolest life I can imagine for myself? Now, to get our health and our life to that point, we need to keep only three things in mind.

First, to escape average we need to do something different from the average person. Here's the raw truth. If we're not where we want to be day to day, with our health, with our body, with our relationships, with our happiness, *then we need to do something different.* Now that may not seem like such an earth shattering statement, because we all know it to be true. Except we don't. We only know it intellectually to be true. Just like we know we're all going to die some day, we don't really believe it. If we did, we would live our lives differently. We would treat our spouse differently. We would enjoy life more and not take it quite as seriously. We would quit jobs we hated sooner, and spend more time doing things we loved. We wouldn't get stressed out nearly as much. It can be tough when we're caught up in the daily grind to remember this.

If I'm not happy with being twenty or thirty pounds overweight, then something about my routine of commute => job => commute => American Idol for three hours has to change. Something has to change. It doesn't need to be big, and it doesn't have to be a lot, but *something* needs to be different. To escape living an average life or average health, we need to stop living like the average person. Of all the principles that have helped me in my life most, it's been this. Want to avoid average anything? Look at what most people you know do every day in that specific aspect of their lives, and make sure your routine looks different.

The principles here go way beyond health. I think you'll see that these basic, daily principles truly will transform your life way bigger than just looking and feeling better than you ever have before. This book will change your life if you let it. In fact, psychologists call exercise a keystone habit, which means that once a person acquires the habits, skills, discipline, etc. to regularly exercise, it spills over into other aspects of their lives. People end up finding themselves calmer, more organized, more resilient, more driven, and happier. Students end up getting higher grades because they begin cultivating crossover habits, discipline, focus, and more – not to mention the mental benefits that come from being healthy.

If you develop the kind of personality where you "show up every day 100%" for your health, imagine what kind of impact that has on your relationship or life when you start living it?

Deliberate living is also the path out of the boring, mundane existence some of us don't want. This book is going to introduce you to a proven system for focusing on your health, *and being deliberate* about what you do each day with it. Naturally, you can apply this to any aspect of your life that "isn't working." Yeah, it's about looking and feeling incredible, better than you ever have before in your life. But it's way bigger than just that. It's about waking up and actually regaining that fire for life. It's about not having poor health that holds you back from doing the things really important to you in life. Do you remember what that felt like?

No?

Hang out with young twenty-something college graduates for a while. They still have that fire in the belly before they got their dreams crushed by the grind. And whether or not they go on to achieve those big dreams is irrelevant – just observe the fire. They're pumped about life. It's exciting. It's an adventure. They can do anything they want. Forget reality for thirty seconds – what would it be like to actually feel like that for a day again?

The way back to that fire you used to have is by *living life deliberately.* These three principles we'll come back to more and more throughout the book. In order to be successful, once and for all, we need to understand these principles and avoid the four "inner" horsemen of the health apocalypse.

Chapter Recap: Getting From Where You Are To Where You Want to Be

☐ **Compound habit interest.** We've been told that compound interest is the eight wonder of the world, but what about compound habit interest? Surprisingly, the biggest life and health transformations come from the smallest actions – just done daily. The "success stories" just chose a few key habits, and made sure they did them each day.

☐ **It's not about moving more and eating less, it's about life.** The reason why being healthy (all the time) is so tough is because we're trying to juggle careers, family life, fun, fulfillment, the poopy diapers of kids, stress, and the inevitable ups and downs of life we can't control – *all at once.* Anyone who says it's about eating less and moving more clearly has no clue.

☐ **Deliberate living is the path back to the health (and honestly, the life) we want.** If we don't think about what we want, it's almost impossible to get what we want. If we merely sit down for a few moments each day to think about the kind of health (and life) we want, it's that much more likely to become a reality.

PART 1

The Four "Inner Horsemen" Of The Health Apocalypse

The Willpower & Discipline Myth: The Little Known Secrets Of Being <u>More</u> Successful With <u>Less</u> Discipline

"I write only when inspiration strikes… fortunately it's every morning at 9 O'clock sharp."

- SOMERSET MORGAN

"So I just counted on my own determination and willpower to adhere to the plans I created for myself. These plans usually consisted of not eating sweets (again, vague!) and working out 4-6 times a week (workout videos, going to the gym, running). The intensity of my determination varied from year to year…at some points, when mustering up new resolve to lose weight, I was convinced that it wouldn't be that hard, while at other times, I felt like I was entering a losing battle from the first day of a new self-prescribed plan. At this point I'm starting to realize that the issue probably goes a lot deeper than eating too much or working out too little. I don't really know where to go from here, but I'm tired of trying the same thing over and over again, and failing at it. I definitely want results (weight loss and

being in shape) but I also would LOVE to figure out what the root problem is that is causing me to have these bad habits."

- JILLIAN, R.

Willpower is a myth. *Huh?* The idea of willpower and discipline being *the* defining character of those who succeed at getting healthy and losing weight – it's a myth. Consider a series of interesting studies done.

In one study, the brain of a chronic emotional eater (binge eater) was scanned with fMRI technology to observe which parts of the brain lit up as the individual person experienced cravings. At the same time, side-by-side, the brain of a cocaine addict was analyzed while he was craving the drug – and guess what the results were? The cravings presented themselves in *identical* portions of the brain – and abundant research now shows[3] that rats will actually put themselves through more pain in the pursuit of *sugar* than they will for *cocaine*. Food is a drug. Literally. There's no debating it. People addicted to eating refined carbohydrates function – almost identically – as drug addicts, where the opioid receptors in the brain are craving more, more, more.

In a separate study, researchers took it even further[4]. Researchers stimulated the portion of the rat's brain with a substance called DAMGO, a synthetic equivalent of an opioid normally produced by the brain. Remember, the opioid receptors are the same ones dealing with food addiction and drug addiction. When the rats were stimulated with this, the rats became hyperactive and stuffed themselves with food.

Here's what's even crazier: these DAMGO stimulated rats didn't drink water more heavily, even when they were thirsty, and it didn't matter if they just ate or were hungry. They all *still* gorged themselves on the food when stimulated. Naturally, the next question that researchers had was if the rats craved any specific forms of food when stimulated. The rats were once again stimulated, and this time given a choice between high fat rat chow and high carb rat chow. Overwhelmingly, the rats preferred the high carb food, *even the rats that normally preferred the high fat food!* Side note: this book is not about eating low carb. I don't recommend it or suggest it as a core strategy. Just throwing that out there. So if food functions almost identically to a drug, and we would *never* tell a drug addict to just "get over their cravings" for cocaine, why on earth do we still think it's just a willpower game, as if there's something wrong with us if we don't "have" willpower?

It's a lot more complex than that. Food is a great part of life when we have a great relationship with it, but food can also become a formidable enemy. Willpower and discipline are losing strategies – especially for those of us that self describe ourselves as *lacking* the aforementioned qualities. If you're a self-described person who "just lacks willpower and motivation" then I know this book will open your mind about what's possible – when you *bypass* this silly old school "grind it out harder" approach. You'll see none of that here. For a long time people talked about willpower and assumed it was *the* "defining" quality of the successful. Discipline. Grit. Fortitude.

Whether you were a successful businessman, super-fit with an insanely non-existent sweet tooth, or someone who just seemed to be successful in everything they did – people assumed it was because of willpower and discipline. Are these critical strategies? Sure! Absolutely. There are loads of successful dieters and financially rich people with iron discipline, who wake up at 4 am, slog through 100 miles, and then grind out a twelve-hour day – and that's just a *normal* day for them.

Does it work? Absolutely. But it works *for them*. What about the other 99.9% of us mortal, human beings who aren't cut from that cloth and run away from the idea of becoming superhuman through sleep deprivation? There's a reason why I hate when these "gurus" say it's all about willpower and discipline. We assume that all people that have gotten somewhere in life or managed to turn their health around are legendary immortals of willpower and discipline that just forced themselves to do more things they hate.

And we assume that supposedly led to their success. Research shows willpower to function like a muscle that has limited power especially as the day goes on[5]. So were those of us "born" without willpower and discipline out of luck? Are we doomed to a life of mediocrity and frail health? Not at all. Willpower is actually not quite as constant and as "built-in" as one might think. Many complex factors affect the strength of our willpower on a daily basis – sleep, stress and nutrition to name a few. Willpower is not exactly the most reliable way to maintain a health and fitness regime or get started. It's too variable. And health is something that *has to be a priority* — so you can't rely upon something as variable as willpower to keep you healthy. So we can either: Create and cultivate massive amounts of willpower (I'll pass), or bypass willpower altogether.

That's when I realized there was a much better "secret." The secret was, in fact, habits, rituals, and cleverly devised systems that anyone can do. We don't fail to stick with our new year's resolution because of lack of willpower or lack of discipline. We aren't lazy, we're not "unmotivated," we just have no idea about how much of our life (and our "success") is governed by our habits.

***

"We are what we repeatedly do. Excellence, then, is not an act, but a habit."

- ARISTOTLE

Everything about us – success, health, happiness, prejudices, friends, aspirations, and outlook on life – is all because of habits and patterns of habitual thinking and acting. Really. We're born with certain things, our environment causes certain things, our life experiences cause certain things – and all of these ingrain certain patterns in our brain.

The cool thing is that just about anything can be un-done (or changed for the better), and the field of neuroplasticity (literally – moldable brain) has shown us that the brain can literally, physically, be re-wired to accommodate new habits and new ways of thinking. [6] That's good news for us.

The "Secrets" of Iron Discipline: Straight From Success Stories

"I feel like I'm just so unmotivated and lazy… I lack willpower and discipline… I don't hold myself accountable… I feel sorry for myself. It's almost embarrassing admitting these things, since

I know what I should be doing, but I just can't get myself to do them."

- NANCY, R., UK

Remember those dozens of interviews I did with people that lost 100+ pounds and kept it off years later, without any calorie counting or fad diets? When we chatted, I was curious as anyone else was and I asked, *"What's your top secret method for discipline?"* And the answers they gave me might surprise you:

"Uhh, method for motivation and discipline?"

"I just… did it."

"If you want it badly enough, you'll find a way." I was pretty disappointed. How was that supposed to help anyone else? Moreover, doesn't that kind of seem like these people were *born* that way? When I dug deeper, here's what I found. When you look at anyone at the top of his or her game, like Olympians, professional authors, athletes and more, *showing up* replaces motivation. Are you starting to see where the idea of *Master the Day* comes from? Motivation is fleeting – some days we feel motivated and other days we don't. Some days we sleep like crap, and all the next day we're lagging and unmotivated.

Some days it's rainy and our mood feels rainy, so we don't want to write a little bit more of that book, go for our walk, or take the time to cook that extra meal. Some days we just flat out have stressful, crappy or hormonal days. And some days… I think you get the picture. Motivation, like willpower, varies *a lot*. People at the top of their game don't rely on it at all.

They rely on one habit: showing up.

***

Showing Up: The Art of Willpower-Free Achievement

"Eighty percent of success is showing up."

- WOODY ALLEN

Something every day. Show up, every single day. Just do something every single day. It doesn't matter if you do five minutes or an hour; just show up every single day to push yourself one step further along the path. Think about the average day most of us dread: Monday. The alarm goes off and shows 6:00 am. Ugh. You slap the snooze button. 6:15, ugh. You slap the snooze button again. 6:30, ugh. Okay, it's time to move. You groggily get out of bed, squinting out of one eye, and then hobble over to the bathroom to brush your teeth and hop in the shower.

You're more tired than usual because Sunday night you stayed up a bit late dreading work the next day and spent some extra time watching a TV show. You make a hasty breakfast, grab some coffee, and you're off. 45 minute commute, ugh. You arrive at the office at 9:06, six minutes late, and catch some flack from the boss.

More ugh.

By the end of the day, *it's been one long Monday*, and at 5:30 pm the only thing you want to do is drive as fast as possible *away* from the office and your coworkers. You're finally home after commuting back from the office, and now you cross the threshold: an important, singular moment that will determine the trajectory of your destiny *forever.* Can you guess what it is? Whether or not to sit down, lose momentum, plop down on the couch with a snack, and remain there – *or* keep the momentum and do something else that might add value to your life. And in that split second life goes in one certain direction – you choose the couch, telling yourself *"it's been a rough Monday at work and I need to relax a bit."* What happened to all that willpower? Where'd the discipline go? Are we really going to start tomorrow, *Tuesday?* I'll tell you what – of the dozens of people I interviewed, *not one* mentioned that they were being insanely disciplined. They used words like "focused" and "being smart with your time" or employing "systems and good time management."

As I dug deeper, I found something even more interesting. Overwhelmingly, the successful people I studied didn't rely on raw willpower. They know that on rainy days, they might not want to go to the gym. But as an Olympian, they need to clock in those 3-6 hours of training a day. As an author, they need to write those 3,000 words a day and edit their drafts. As an artist, they have to paint no matter how they feel, or else they don't eat. Consider the training regime of Michael Phelps, featured in Charles Duhigg's book, book *The Power of Habit*:

> *"What Bowman could give Phelps, however – what would set him apart from other competitors – were habits that would make him the strongest mental swimmer in the pool. He didn't need to control every aspect of Phelps's life. All he needed to do was target a few specific habits that had nothing to do with swimming and everything to do with creating the right mindset. He designed a series of behaviours that Phelps could use to become calm and focused before each race, to find those tiny advantages that, in a sport where victory can come in milliseconds, would make all the difference. When Phelps was a teenager, for instance, at the end of each practice, Bowman would tell him to go home and "watch the videotape. Watch it before you go to sleep and when you wake up." The videotape wasn't real. Rather, it was a mental visualization of the perfect race. Each night before falling asleep and each morning after waking up, Phelps would imagine himself jumping off the blocks and, in slow motion, swimming flawlessly. He would imagine the wake behind his body, the water dripping off his lips as his mouth cleared the surface, what it would feel like to rip off his cap at the end. He would lie in bed with his eyes shut and watch the entire competition, the smallest details, again and again, until he knew each second by heart."[7]*

This is the power of rituals, routines, and most of all – *habits*. Not massive willpower, but the exact opposite: tiny things we do *every* day, *without fail*. That's what's standing between where you are, and where you want to be. *Showing up* is more important (no matter how small) than developing insane, superhero levels of self-control. The more we tell ourselves, "I just don't have that much discipline and willpower" the more we attempt to give ourselves a legitimate excuse to quit.

When we reframe it, remove willpower and discipline from the picture, and instead focus on key tiny habits, routines, rituals, and just *showing up*, no matter how small, that's when big things start happening.

Chapter Recap: The Willpower & Discipline Myth

☐ **Food is a drug.** It shares the same neural pathways that cocaine and other opiates share; yet we would never tell a drug addict to *will* their way out of cravings. So why do we tell people just to use more willpower?

☐ **Something every day philosophy.** Willpower and discipline help, there's no doubt about it. But an even easier philosophy is the "something every day" concept. Just do one thing each day to push you closer to where you want to be - and don't obsess over the goal – obsess over the process. We often underestimate the power of just doing a little bit each day (even if it seems like nothing), and the huge impact it can have on your life after a few months or a year.

☐ **Olympians use routines, habits, and daily rituals.** Rather than being iron-willed, Olympians have rules like "I have to show up every day" or "I have to train Monday-Saturday." Almost all of them have daily rituals and routines too – like work, you just show up. Some days you want to, some you don't, but you do it anyway. Feelings vary and willpower does too.

The Silver Bullet: Magical Weight Loss Pills Found on Unicorn Poop in the Amazon (& Other Shortcuts)

"Please, PLEASE Alex, before you go, can you just answer one question?" she asked.

"Sure," I said. "What is it?"

"What's *the secret*? What's the magic bullet? Can you just give me that *one* piece of advice that would change it all? Is it carbs? Is it fat? Just give me the answer! Spare me the pain…" She pleaded. Stacy was on a brief call with me to assess her current health, lifestyle, and goals. And although I was totally empathetic to her situation, I couldn't help but feel a bit guilty when I cringed and said, "The biggest secret is that there is no secret – it's just daily habits, applied over time."

Her heart sank. What else was I supposed to tell her though? Everyone wants a secret – and the sad truth is that smart marketers, big companies, and more unethical folks will *gladly* sell us it. It makes total sense, right? Who doesn't want to get fitter, healthier, happier, richer, *faster*? Uhh, *I do*! This is why diets will sell like mad, and will always continue to sell – forever – as long as people are overweight, feel like crap and want to get rid of it quickly.

A diet implies that you just "follow these 3 easy steps" and you'll get the outcome you want – no struggle required, and not much time required. It's really quite brilliant in theory, but it's horrible in reality. Anyone who has dieted (most of us?) has realized this is anything *but* the truth. We tend to forget *The Key: The Narrative* + tiny daily habits = your dream body, and amazing health.

Let me show you what that looks like in action, and why the looking for silver bullet, waiting for the big break, and waiting for the alignment of the planets is fatal to success.

Anatomy of A Life Gone Haywire

"I just don't even know how I got here… It feels like I woke up in someone else's life. I'm 42, forty pounds overweight, I hate my job, my health is terrible, and I can barely drag myself out of bed in the morning. But here's the frustrating part… I don't even know how I got here. I feel like I just woke up in a nightmare, in a bad dream, in someone else's life. I didn't think it would ever end up like this… I'm just so lost. In my 20s I was so ambitious. I had all these dreams of traveling the world, writing a book, starting a movement and doing something I loved. My health is just one part of this nightmare. How did this even happen?"

- Confused coaching client

What we often don't realize is that our current life is a reflection of thousands of tiny actions that we've been engaging in every single day, for hundreds or thousands of days. The problem is that one day we wake up, look at ourselves in the mirror (or our bank account, or our happiness, or our marriage), and go "Whoa, what happened?" We act as if it happened over night. But did it really? Of course not.

I've talked to a lot of people that can describe this surreal feeling of time passing and waking up in someone else's life. It's beyond scary. And usually it happens to all of us at some point in life. We hit that financial crossroads our 20s or 30s when we haven't learned about personal finance, we hit the health crossroads in our 30s and 40s after the years of neglect and partying pile up, and sometimes we hit the relationship crossroads after a decade or more of being married. But the truth is that this magical event didn't happen by itself – and it didn't happen just from one isolated incident.

It happened because of things we did every single day, whether or not we thought about what we were doing. It happened because of tiny daily habits. Habits that were so tiny, so negligible, so imperceptible that at the time it didn't matter that we were making them – so we didn't pay attention. Once we realize this key concept, everything in life changes. We'll really get that there really is no one, magical silver bullet to fix the problem. We'll no longer think that just "ONE" thing will solve all our problems.

So let's take a look at a few examples now, before talking about how this affects our health.

Tiny Daily Habits & The Story of John's Relationship:

John comes home one day and finds a note from his wife, and none of his children in the house. *"We're staying at Sally's,"* it says. He feels that sick feeling in his stomach as his intuition gets the meaning. He's crushed. He has *no idea* how this could have happened? Where did he go wrong? What did he do wrong? John's truly at a loss for words.

Well the truth was that *what he didn't do* was just as important as what he did do. Because at the end of the day – John engaged in hundreds of tiny habits – habits that either pushed him closer to his goals, or further away from his goals. In the grand scheme of things, we're either improving or getting worse – it just happens so imperceptibly slow that we don't realize it. It's like the changing of the seasons. It seems to take forever to get to summer, and then gradually the days get warmer and longer. One day, it's 85 degrees and we're sitting on the beach loving our life somewhere warm. And gradually the days get shorter and the air gets colder – but it seems like "one day" we just wake up, the trees are bare, and the crisp winter winds are blowing through town.

"It seems like summer was barely here!" we say *every single year*. That's how life is – change is constant, but often so slow we don't see it – we only notice it as years elapse. The aging process works the same way. Back to John: he engaged in hundreds of tiny habits every single day, which either got him *closer* to the great marriage he wanted, or pushed him away from his spouse. John just wasn't self aware enough to pay attention to his choices in the moment, like the following.

Out of 30 basketball games for his son Billy, he missed 22 of them. That's a 26% attendance rate. He also didn't realize that because of the stress at his job, he rushed out of the house, never said thank you to his amazing wife that cooked him a nutritious breakfast and made him coffee, and once he returned home late at night all he did was complain. He was too absorbed in his own projects, his own career, to remember to ask her how *her* day was (hint: it was bad, but he never asked, so she never told.) He often felt bad about these things, but he rationalized them, saying, "Oh, it's just once. It's just a stressful workweek, I can go back to being a great husband after, I just need to focus on this for now. I'll attend more of Billy's games too – I've only missed one this month."

And now, an even bigger problem arose: He rationalized this with his health too. "I know I've been going out to business lunches a lot recently, but I'll start wrapping this up closer to the new year." Because he found himself eating out for lunch and getting some alcohol for his business meetings each week, he was adding an extra 500-1000 calories a day to his lifestyle. No big deal in the short run, but here's what his life and health looks like after five years.

Flash forward 5 years. John's "oh it's only missing a game once" now looks like this: 8/30 Games per year, x 5 years = 40 games he went to out of, 150. 25% there. Failing grades. Making his wife feel appreciated and loved, (104 days out of 365 in a year), x 5 years, = 28% attendance rate. That's also failing. Finally, because of his business lunches (a beer or two, and a pasta dish), he added an extra 3500 calories a week to his diet. As a result, he gained weight slowly (imperceptibly at first), but steadily.

Over a few months he noticed that his belt was a bit tighter, but it wasn't that dramatic and it wasn't really a big issue. He gained about a pound (let's say half a pound a week) at that rate, and to be honest, even after 2.5 months, that was only 5 pounds. Not really noticeable. But after the first year? 25 pounds. And after year two? 50 pounds. And year three? 75 pounds. By year five, John was borderline clinically obese, almost 275 pounds at a height of 6' 2", and had all the associated problems dominating his life. Acid reflux, constipation, high blood pressure, constantly being winded, waking up at night, and his stress levels were unbearable. Food became a close friend more than ever before – now he needed it.

One day, at the peak of John's collapse, he just quit. He gave up. He threw in the towel. First he had his health and weight problems. Now his wife left him. His kids hated him. And to top it all off, he realized that *he worked this hard* for them the entire time; he just didn't do a good job understanding how his daily choices (or lack of choices) affected his future.

"How did it ever get to this point?"

***

Five years ago, life was great for John. He had a loving wife, amazing kids, decent health (no big issues), and life was stressful but balanced and fun. Now he had no wife, his kids hated him, and he was on the verge of a major health breakdown.

"Why is this happening to me?! Someone help me!" he would cry sometimes at night. But John did this to himself – he just didn't realize it. He did this to himself because he made choices (with or without realizing it) that led him down the path he's on now. There were no coincidences, no bad luck, no karma, just choices. And the good thing, or the scary thing is, we have the same power. We have the power to make these great choices, or the power to make choices that will punish and cripple us in the long run. It sounds like some heavy stuff, and it can be, but it's worth re-iterating as many times as possible.

The Tale of Chronically Poor Chris

One of my friends, who we'll call *Chronically Poor Chris*, is, well, always poor. The sad thing is that Chris has a pretty good job – at 27 he makes about $60,000, so after taxes he takes home a little under $4,000 per month. He's going steady with his girlfriend, but he doesn't have a mortgage to pay, just rent, and has no large expenses. Technically he should be pretty secure and putting a lot of money away.

But Chris (because he realizes that he has such a strong salary for his age), doesn't understand this *Psychology + Little Daily Habits* idea. He rationalizes overspending easily, "Dude, I make so much anyway," and is in denial about how much he spends, saying, "I only eat out once per day." As a result, when he gets paid, he spends. By 30, even though Chris was making an enormous amount of money for someone his age, he had a savings account with $15.26 in it. Yeah, *$15 dollars*. And that was because his silly money market savings account carried over the pennies from the past five years.

Let me tell you the story of another person now: Saver Sally. Sally has been stashing $200 a month away since she was 27, half into a Roth IRA and half into a generic savings account for emergencies. Despite the fact that she only makes $35k as a social worker, by 30 she has saved:

* $7,200 total
* $3,600 in her IRA
* $3,600 in her emergency fund

We make the same decisions with our finances every single day – whether or not we make the decision consciously. It doesn't really require any more effort - it just requires different choices. This is a big theme here: better health doesn't necessarily require massive effort, discipline, willpower and huge time investments. It just requires that we change our fundamental choices, because those choices become our habits.

Sarah, The Most Unlucky Marketing Manager On the Planet

Sarah is a 26-year-old marketing manager at a new startup in her local area. She had an incredibly tough time finding a job out of college, and now that she has one, she's been thanking her lucky stars. But unfortunately, just a few short years later after *finally* becoming stable she gets fired. No job. No income.

"Why am I always so unlucky?" she says. That day, the cashier at the local coffee shop spills some hot coffee on her.

"Great, more bad luck." On the way home, she rear-ends the car in front of her, wracking up another $500 bill.

"Can this day get any worse?" Why, yes it can. A few short months later, her mom is hospitalized with a chronic condition and pulls in a whopping $50,325 medical bill. And as all these things occur in Sarah's life, her life begins to spiral out of control, and she goes into a deep depression. Every time her friends see her, she's always complaining about her stupid coworkers at her new local minimum wage job. "I work with such lazy idiots," she constantly says. She's always talking about the fire and brimstone on TV, the latest conspiracy about how the government is trying to keep her down, and about how life is all one big cosmic game where we're the ants, and the supreme creator is some kind of bully with a magnifying glass. Over time even her friends stop hanging out with her because of her negativity.

Now, she's *really* at rock bottom.

***

Was Sarah really that unlucky? Or did she really just not realize that the daily tiny habits she was engaging in were leading her down the road to ruin? She didn't realize that her gossip talking and complaining at her minimum wage job was what got her fired from her marketing manager job. She didn't realize that the reason she had coffee spilled on her on that horrible day was because she was in her head thinking of all the things she wanted to say to her boss, and she bumped the person next to her. She didn't realize that she rear-ended the car because she was yet again rushing – another bad daily habit.

Finally, she lost all her friends because of her constantly negative, fire and brimstone talk. And all this time, she thought the world was teaming up on her, trying to ruin her life. As if it had some cosmic agenda to bully individual people and make their lives a wreck. But what Sarah didn't know, if Sarah watched the tape of her own life filmed in third person, was that there were a few systems and psychological habits holding her back. There were a few repetitive routines causing most of the misfortune in her life.

Is this an overly example dramatic? Yeah, of course! But we often wander through life suffering from the same symptoms: poor health, the same flawed relationships, not enough money, and unhappiness – for the same reasons. We don't understand the tiny daily habits (the emotional and psychological systems) occurring in our life that are creating the outcomes we see. This is what I wish I knew ten years ago – the real secret to success.

If only people understood that health, happiness, wealth, fulfillment, and yes, weight loss, are not about quantum leaps, big breaks, super fast progress, deadlines and hard goals. If only people could understand that our current life is a reflection of the past 10,000 choices we had made. It's about whether or not we said "I love you" to our spouse over the past 5 years. It's about whether we decided to attend the sports games of our children, or the piano recitals, or making sure we're were home for little play dates. It's about whether or not we decide to have "just one" Frappuccino each day.

Whether we decided to use food as a way to combat stress at the office – or whether we decided to go for a walk around the block or relax with a friend. Whether we decided to wake up 30 minutes earlier and cook a great, nutritious breakfast and relax, or whether we slept 30 minutes later and rushed around like a nut job each morning.

The 5 Most Important Seconds of Our Life - The Power of Choice

The most incredible force in the universe is quite simple. It doesn't matter if you're male or female, white or black, young or old. It doesn't care how many times you've failed before or how many successes you've already had.

It's the power of choice.

It doesn't discriminate – if you aren't happy where you are right now with the state of your health, your weight, your finances, or your happiness – you can change it *right now*. Yes, starting today. All of these little things are just the result of snowballs that grow larger and larger every day as we make choices that support progress and growth, or choices that dig us deeper into the hole. You know that whole "excellence is not an act, but a habit" quote? Here's what that really looks like in action - with a tiny habit.

Let's say over the period of three weeks, we cultivate the habit of stress eating less. So maybe we're eating just 200 calories less a day - because we're avoiding those late night Oreos. Seems like an insignificant habit, right? Just avoiding a couple Oreos a night. But that results in 1400 fewer calories a week, or about half a pound lost. After week one, there's almost no progress. A half-pound. Could be a fluke. After two weeks, still no progress. A pound. Almost nothing. But here's where those who succeed keep going, and those who fail stop.

After 4 weeks: 2 pounds lost.

After 8 weeks: 4 pounds lost.

After 12 weeks: 6 pounds lost.

After 1/2 a year: 12 pounds lost.

After a year: 24 pounds lost.

Now, realistically weight loss is *not* this easily predicted by math. But this is the reason why so few of us succeed. Imagine if you just looked at the first 4 weeks and decided to quit? Two pounds is nothing. You can't see it. You can lose more than two pounds of water weight on a hot summer day running around outside. But after you keep doing this one tiny habit, which takes virtually no time, after a year you are in a different body altogether.

Pretend you can predict the future. So you're sitting up there in the sky, looking down on your future – the next 12 months. Imagine doing work every day, and not seeing any visible results for eight weeks: two months. Most people have already quit. Even twelve weeks in: six pounds is right around where people start noticing a big difference. But was it really worth waiting three *months?* Now zoom ahead even further: half a year, twelve pounds lost.

That's substantial.

And that took about 100 days to get there. This "100 day rule" is the lense I encourage people to view progress through. Whatever habit you're trying to cultivate for your health, can you see results in thirty days? Sure! Realistically, the 100-day window is a much better one. And don't forget a very important thing. This is all the result of just spending *five minutes* a day doing one thing, and then being patient and letting time work its magic.

And every day we have the power of choice. During each week, it begins on Sunday night. Do you have a game plan for breakfast Monday morning? Are you getting up a few minutes earlier so you don't have to run around like a madman? And then lunch at the office – are you going out to a business lunch and ordering the big bowl of pasta with a tiramisu dessert and a glass of wine, or are you getting the baked salmon with rice and greens, and drinking tea, water or one less glass of wine?

And then your commute home – are you sitting there stressing in traffic, sending your stress hormones off the charts, or are you listening to something inspiring that can change your life in a half hour? And then in the evening – are you driving home exhausted, and plopping down on the couch to relax or are you taking that 10-minute walk which is going to dramatically improve your mood? And then how you interact with your spouse and your kids – are you letting yourself lose your cool, are you nagging and repeating the same things, are you yelling and pulling your hair out or trying something new?

At the end of the day we all have the same gift- the power of choice – which is the gift to *transform everything in our life* in a single moment. In one instant, you can't see it, but everything changes. This is how you can change the entire trajectory of your life in less than five seconds.

Why There Is No Silver Bullet, Magical Formula, Or Hidden Secret Awaiting Discovery

There is no one big aha moment for most people. There is no perfect time to get healthy, decide life has to change, or embark on creating the "new you." There's no such thing as the perfect time – there are only daily habits, and the sooner we cultivate them, the sooner we arrive at where we want to be (and who we want to be). The stars won't magically align, and your zodiac chart won't say " this is the year, begin! It'll all fall into place effortlessly!"

That's a luxury that most people don't get, and can't afford. For most people, life pushes us and teaches us with nudges – little aches here or there, indigestion that keeps cropping up, a spouse that seems a bit distant. These things are easy to ignore if you choose to, or if you're moving too fast to see them. Sometimes we're too busy chasing other goals (success, fun, etc.) and we deliberately don't pay attention. But by far, there is one big myth standing between us, and the body, health, and dreams that we want: the myth of the big break, the perfect time, or the silver bullet.

Just like the woman I told you about earlier, who pleaded with me desperately, *"Alex, please, what's the secret? Can you share just one piece of advice that will change my life?"* many of my own students and clients often pray for this too. And the psychology behind this is why so often we fail to live the lives we want. Think about it: believing in the big break implies this: *"Once I find the perfect formula and system, my health and weight loss will rapidly come to me, and I'll achieve my goals quickly with the aid of this silver bullet."*

And what happens? We wait for the silver bullet. We wait. And we wait. And we wait some more. And we keep on waiting for the silver bullet to show up and make it all easy. And then we do nothing, because it doesn't show up. And time flies by: summer arrives, summer goes away, fall arrives, and then it gets colder. Winter arrives, and then suddenly it seems like it's the New Year again. "Wow, a year sure passed fast!"

But are we any closer to the health, the body, the dreams, the life that we want? Not at all - we were too busy waiting for the "silver bullet" to arrive.

I read a story recently about a kid who was constantly told he was special, incredible, brilliant and would go on to do "amazing things" with his life. In fact, all his classmates voted that he was most likely to do something amazing in the next few years. Flash-forward about ten years, some time around his high school reunion. A random interviewer snaps a picture of him, and asks him about his "story." He talks about how everyone said he was sure to do "great things" in the world way back in high school, about ten years ago. And here was his exact response:

> *"Everyone told me, Juan, that you're going to do amazing, big things in the world. But I spent so much time looking for what my big thing was, that ten years later, I passed up on a lot of other "small things" that could've amounted to big things if I took action and wasn't waiting for the big break. I feel like I missed so much…"*

It's not coming. Remember the power of 1% better. The quickest path between where we are and where we want to be is simple: our daily habits and choices. The sooner we begin, the sooner that snowballs into an incredible, vibrant, fulfilling life – magnitudes larger than just being healthy and fit.

Why Silver Bullets Are Everywhere

Don't you think if silver bullets existed, more people would be using them? If some revolutionary shortcut truly existed that worked for so many people, don't you think you would've heard about it? Let me let you in on a little secret: the only industries that successfully sell silver bullets (make money, weight loss, manifesting your dreams) sell them because they know *that people know the truth but don't want to accept it* and do the work. Think about your own personal life experience. Who are some of your friends that you know are super healthy or fit?

Do they regularly do some kind of physical activity? (Probably). Do they regularly do some kind of healthy eating? (Probably). Do they actually make *health* a focus of their life? (Probably). So why isn't your successful, healthy friend buying some of these silver bullets?

Now, who are some of your friends that are really financially secure and set. Did they get it over night? Unless your friend inherited it, chances are you remember him or her working long hours, right? Chances are, you remember her missing events, you remember her traveling, and you remember her not always being there for her family. You probably remember her reading business books, listening to audiotapes, and attending conferences and seminars.

In other words, s*he paid the price*. She did the work. So let me share something: there isn't just one revolutionary piece of advice that will forever make it easy to lose weight, keep it off, and stay healthy forever (except the ideas in this book, obviously!) That's because tips, tactics, formulas, and diets change and work for us all differently: the only constant is us. There is no one magical diet. There is no one magical health tip (like going low carb, or going low fat). There is no magical supplement (I know deep down you *know* a supplement can't magically transform your body by itself – even if it *was* found on unicorn poop in South America).

There is no big break. The stars will rarely align, the clouds will seldom part, and a giant, cosmic slap in the face (with the 'secret') will never arrive. At least for most people it doesn't. Once you understand this, you'll realize that *anything* in life you want is possible – the dream body, the happiness, the stress-free living, and yes any and all financial goals. Because you, and your current life (the one you're waking up to today), is just a reflection of the habits, and the choices you have made or avoided over the past few years (or decades). And the choices or habits you *avoid* are often just as important as the ones you engage in every day.

Lottery Winners, Tiny Daily Habits and The Lies
of a Better Life

In 2004 Sharon Tirabassi was a single mother on welfare, before winning the Ontario Lottery for over $10 million dollars. Almost overnight she went from being on welfare and taking the local city bus, to buying a big house, four cars, exotic trips, lavish clothing, and handing out money left and right to friends and family. She flew out of the country when she wanted, stayed where she wanted, had a fully customized Cadillac Escalade, and lots more.

Life was good. There was one problem though: nine years later, by 2013, she was totally broke. Actually, she was *beyond* broke: she was back riding the public bus, working part-time, and living in a house she was renting to make ends meet. How is this even possible?

"You've got to be joking me! This person must be seriously dense to burn ten million dollars like that… I would do so much better if I won the lotto." It might be easy to think that, but hear me out. Lots of "financial coaches" will tell you that it's about the individual's "financial blueprint." In other words these people didn't have the character or personality to know what to do with this, so they reverted back to their "blueprint" which obviously wasn't $10 or $25 million.

A person who was historically a saver and knew how to hold on to money probably would not have gone broke and into debt like many lottery winners do. And that's because their *habits* and character were aligned with saving, frugality, and being very careful with money. Here's my point.

The exact same is true with how we approach health and weight loss. If we don't change our habits, our behaviors, our mindset, and *The Narrative*, nothing changes – ever – no matter how many diets we try, coaches we hire, and pills we take. That includes the whole "big break" theory. If we keep believing in the silver bullet, the big break, the stars aligning, what diet or plan will help us?

Nothing will change unless we do. This is why so often we change diets or plans, and yet again – as always – end up back at *square one* with the *exact same goals* we had just a few months ago or last year's new year. We keep changing what we put in (what information), without changing our own blueprint: our daily habits, our behavior, our psychology and our approach. The silver bullet, big break, stars aligning is a myth. The longer we wait, the longer it takes to get to where we want to be. The great health, the great body, the great *life* we want, is just on the other side of thousands of tiny daily choices we make – and the sooner we begin, the sooner we arrive.

Chapter Recap: Silver Bullets

☐ **There is no magical silver bullet.** There is no perfect system for all of us, there is no magic pill, no silver bullet – just daily habits applied over time. The more we wait for the silver bullet, the longer it takes to look and feel incredible.

☐ **Woke up in someone else's life?** That feeling of "how did I get here?" originates because we didn't pay attention to our daily life, we weren't living deliberately, and we we're conscious of what we wanted – and whether our choices were bringing us closer to them or further away.

☐ **Choices each day are how we get back to the health & life we want.** The way *back* to where we want to be is the opposite: living deliberately, thinking about what we want, and then clarifying what daily actions are going to get us there.

I Came, I Saw, I… Failed (Getting Over Perfectionism & Being Way Too Serious)

"I was doing great all week, but last Friday it was my close friend's birthday so we all went out. I didn't want to be that one awkward person not drinking anything, not eating pizza, not having a bite of the cake, not having a margarita, so I caved. A few minutes in I realized, "Well, I've derailed my progress thus far, and pretty much undid all my week's work. Better just enjoy myself! It was a nightmare. Too many drinks. Too much junk. Too much. And now, Saturday morning I don't even see the point of trying again. I mean, I lost. I've been beat. All the hard work I did each day I just poured down the drain. Should I bother even starting over?"

How often do we get stuck feeling like every little mess up is catastrophic, and every little win is, well, *little*? A couple years back I was desperately trying to become a regular meditator. I was a pretty neurotic perfectionist (I still am), so truth be told, I did a good job of avoiding sharing my failures with people, and always wanted to stick with the plan 100% while trying to look better than other people.

Most of the time, this usually led me to anxiety so bad I would have half a dozen mini nervous breakdowns a week. In any case, the funny thing was that I *liked* the habit of meditating. I started pretty early in life, when I was around twelve years old, and I liked it ever since. I guess I had this romantic idea that attaining enlightenment and not going insane 24/7 would be easy: It was supposed to be about going with the flow, relaxing, taking it easy, right?

Wrong.

I quickly realized just how human I really was. Although I enjoyed meditating, and I wanted (needed) the benefits it provided, I just couldn't get myself to do it *every day*. I knew that just about anything you do seven days a week produced a pretty measurable impact in your life, and I needed sanity. The thing was that I didn't have much trouble once I sat down on the cushion in my bedroom. And I wasn't bored, frustrated, or hating the entire process.

So it was quite puzzling as to why it was so difficult for me to actually sit on the damn cushion. I would be a mini Buddha for a day and go for a solid 30-40 minutes, and then the next day it would be zero because I realized it was six at night and I hadn't sat down yet. Or Thursday I would do it and Friday I decided that I wanted pizza and beer rather than enlightenment.

Inevitably, once I chose pizza and beer over enlightenment a few times, I started feeling pretty guilty.

"Dude, you're doing this for *your self*. So why aren't you actually doing it?" The more I messed up, the more I wondered why I even bothered trying. "If I can't do at least 30 minutes a day, it's not worth doing because I won't see dramatic results," I kept telling myself.

But was it really *true*? We can easily get stuck thinking that if we mess up today, it's not even worth trying tomorrow. But if we pause for a second, we can see that this is just our emotions cropping up, *The Narrative* getting loud, reminding us that "we're a failure." We'll talk more about *The Narrative* in part two. But is it really true? If we stuck with all our tiny healthy habits all week, and then Friday rolls around and we have a few too many beers or glasses of red wine, did it *really* ruin the progress of the entire week? And it is really black or white? Did you really *hit your goals* or plain old fail? I wish someone would've told me sooner that I was a perfectionist: the worst kind.

How Perfectionism Prevents Success

It wasn't until quite a few years later, when I saw this trait manifest in many other aspects of my life (my relationship, my finances, pretty much any sport I ever tried) that I began to investigate. Do these sound like you?

First, we tend to be overly rigid. To the perfectionist, everything has to go just as we have planned. We need *control*. If we don't have control, our neat, pretty, perfect little plans fly out the window and we go nuts. It just doesn't work. Despite the fact that we understand that life is about change and we can't possibly control everything, we don't want to hear it or acknowledge it. Nope!

Next, we have an extreme fear of failure – that we won't admit. We hold ourselves to unrealistic standards and have unrealistic goals, and we tie our self worth to how well we achieve our goals. Failure is obviously the scariest thing possible, because first of all, failure is catastrophic to perfectionists – even a small failure to the average person is a massive meltdown to us. Life is either success *or* failure. We're either the best, or we're not even going to bother trying. It's stick to the diet 7/7 days, or just give up and quit.

This extreme fear of failure prevents us from learning: where failure is necessary. We're so terrified by the idea that we may not be perfect – that we might not achieve 100% of the goal – that we often avoid things that even have a tiny, remote chance of failure. This is a huge problem. Imagine if a child who hadn't learned how to walk yet was a perfectionist?

"Oh man, I'll never learn to walk!!! I quit!! This is such a waste of my time!" It's laughable, right? But 100% of children are successful. Ponder that. Every single child learns to walk, despite failing for days, weeks and months – and they never lose that spirit. Can you see how harmful perfectionism is to actually *succeeding?*

Third, we procrastinate, because it has to be just right. A close friend of the "fear of failure" thing is procrastination. Obviously, if you think you're going to fail, and failure means you're emotionally going to get crushed or severely depressed, you'll procrastinate because it's been built into a huge beast. Here's the problem: we tend to procrastinate on even small things when we're perfectionists.

Because we've built up failure to be such a big, nasty thing, small stuff like missing one day of eating right, or one day of walking, or one day of meditation is a big deal. And if you think you're going to fail again, we drag ourselves and think, "mehh, I'll get around to it soon."

We also put way too much pressure on ourselves. "I'm going to make this happen *no matter what!"* is a statement I frequently tell myself. I tell myself I'll stay up all night, work when all my friends are having fun, spend my weekends in a cafe working, and do whatever it takes to get to where I want to be. Obviously this insane amount of rigidity and self-pressure can make us pop. What I've personally noticed is that I don't often hold other people to the standard I hold myself to. I won't expect a certain person to put in effort, but I'll expect myself to put in the effort of the #1 achiever. The self-pressure we put on ourselves sometimes leads to meltdowns, breakdowns, panic attacks, or just overall anxiety. "Must perform, must achieve, must be perfect" is how the story tends to go. But what happens when that doesn't work out?

We tend to think in "all or nothing" terms. When I think back in my life, I didn't start anything I knew I couldn't become one of the best at. In my major in college, Biology, the bonus courses that I took I worked overtime to prove I was the best. But there's a dark side: we often want to *look the best* – even if we aren't. So we want to look good, be special, and feel important. When I started Judo and other hobbies I noticed the same thing. If I got beat, my interest in the sport waned. I realized that I just wanted to look good and craved the feeling of "being special."

How often do we start some kind of health regime, and we do *great* the first week, and then Friday rolls around and it's a friend's birthday or some kind of social event. One of our friends says, "oh, just live a little" so we cave, enjoy the night, and then have that massive guilt the next day. Did I just mess up all my hard work? Why bother even starting up? I ruined it all...This is classic perfectionism.

We also tend to get depressed when the goal isn't met. Succeeding at achieving our insanely huge, unrealistic goals is great when it works. But for perfectionists, it sucks way worse when it doesn't work. We beat ourselves up for months or years. Some of us quit passion pursuits for life. You can see this lots in top athletes that are on a winning streak, and once they lose once, they quit like a little kid. If they can't be the best, they won't play the game. Some successful people that have success streaks without any failures commit suicide when they finally *do* fail. Since we "live" for achieving and pushing ourselves to that next level, if we don't get there, we stop.

We also tend to have low self-esteem if we rarely live up to our own expectations. And since our self-esteem is closely tied to our self-achievement, when we don't achieve the things we like, as big as we'd like, or as fast as we'd like, we're crushed. We begin hating ourselves. We doubt if our dream or goal is even possible or realistic. And over time as we internalize the story of "I'm a failure," it can become a reality as we get more and more depressed and doubtful. But ironically, being a perfectionist makes failing *much more likely*.

Wait, don't I *want* to be ambitious with my goal setting? Don't I want to reach for some of these crazy goals, and aim for transforming my life in one year? Totally – but there's a difference between growing and getting better, and being a perfectionist which ruins your ability to progress without stress. Consider the following: Perfectionism is linked to obesity. One study found significant positive associations with obesity, weight issues and binge eating.[8] What's worse was that the participants reported more feelings of powerlessness, more impulsivity, a higher degree of perfectionism and lower self esteem the worse they experienced these episodes.

Perfectionism is also linked to eating disorders. Another study found that perfectionism is linked to obesity and binge eating in women.[9] Whereas the people in the study analyzed a couple key characteristics like media exposure, weight stereotypes, "fat talk," emotional eating, and more, these were *all* worsened by perfectionism. And ultimately, perfectionism is linked to failure and low self esteem. One study done on 149 students found that when they failed or had a rough day, they were more likely to blame themselves and not cope very well with the "failure."[10] So at the end of the day, it might seem like it makes sense to be that person that inspires the room with your huge goal, but if you know you're a perfectionist, here's what you can do about it (to ensure long term success).

Obviously, no list of 5, 7, 9 or 21 tactics can fix a deeply ingrained personality trait. For me it's taken years of practice and regular work on it. Chances are, you won't just wake up one day and not take life so seriously. Chances are you won't wake up one day and stop being so competitive, stop setting huge, unrealistic goals, and stop beating yourself up. But for us, it takes an overall mindset shift – a totally different approach to life. And here's what I mean.

First, Remember The Unbeatable Child's Mind

Remember my analogy about kids? I've heard this example a few times, and it instantly resonated with me. Kids are born resilient. They're born bouncy. They fall down, get hurt, cry, and then get back up. They have to otherwise they don't survive. Kids struggle to learn to talk for years, and make thousands of tiny mistakes before finally beginning to articulate their first sentences in life. And ultimately, the most relevant example is how kids learn to walk or ride a bike.

When a child first crawls between 9-12 months, that's all they do. But then they push the envelope. And they try standing. They always fall down. And they try again. And they fall down. And eventually, they hang onto a piece of furniture or mommy's hand, and they begin to stand. The next step is learning to walk. This one is a lot less fun because if you can't walk, you fall down, and you often fall down hard. Up they go, down they go, up they go, and down they go.

Can you imagine a child perfectionist? "Man, I'm never going to be able to walk! forget this!" Imagine if this one particular child quit. Can you imagine how ridiculous that would be if they just looked around another room full of kids the same age learning to walk? Some were already there walking easily, some were still falling, some were still crawling – but all of them learned to walk eventually. And children have this inherently playful attitude, which is no coincidence. Playfulness is adaptive, and makes you much more likely to learn, succeed, and grow ultimately.

Perfectionism inherently is deadly – it doesn't lead to growth and improvement. It's against the way of nature – being playful, learning, not taking life so seriously. Eventually, every child is successful at learning how to walk. They forget the goal for a time, laugh, have fun, and keep trying until they get there. And they all do.

Have a Goal, But Ignore it Day-To-Day

It's important to have the goal, there's no doubt about it. But what's more important is that we focus on the day-to-day, a concept that I call *Master the Day*. Especially for perfectionists, we are *extremely likely* to become so goal obsessed that we let the present vaporize before our eyes. "Nothing matters until I get there," is kind of the unspoken rule for us. Unfortunately, this is what often drives us insane. Ridiculous goal setting without enjoying the process is what leads to that "Holy crap… how did I get here?" feeling that some of us wake up to in our 40s and 50s. Here's what I'd suggest.

For starters, stop doing the things you hate to get healthy, and instead, focus on things you enjoy. I realize that having fun in life sounds crazy. But here's the basic idea: Chances are, you're not going to do stuff you hate, even if you can get yourself to do it in the short run. So if you hate running, don't run. Go do yoga or do a zumba class. Take a course in martial arts. Do something else. Habits more aligned with your interests are ones you are going to keep doing.

Ignore Achievement & Focus on Progress

One of the toughest things I've struggled with is fighting the feeling of "needing to achieve the goal" that I set for myself. *I have to lose those 30 pounds. I have to get my energy, sleep through the night, and meditate a half hour a day.* There's a bigger problem though: the more we emphasize the goal, the *less* we emphasize the process. And this is flat out a very fast road to unhappiness. I have an alternative: Overcome the feeling of craving success by just *showing up every day.*

Many of us perfectionists are achievers – we have to do something every day to feel productive, like we've taken a step towards our goal. But focusing on the goal can lead to anxiety. So here's a principle that has dramatically changed my life. Just do something every day. That's your goal for the day. Whether it's a 5 minute walk, three minutes of meditation, or ten minutes of yoga, as long as you do something every day you can cross off the goal from your list for the day – *guilt free.*

Remember That Getting Derailed Temporarily Doesn't Derail Your Progress

I hear things like this a lot: *"I did so well for a week, and then on the weekend I went out with friends for a special occasion, ate like crap, felt so guilty the next day, and then decided that I messed up the entire week's progress, so I quit. I repeat this over and over and over."* Be logical. Let's say you made 75% of your dinner tonight. Obviously it's not "ready" – but you still have 75% of a meal. It's not like you're going to starve or go hungry. 3/4 of the plate is filled. The inner perfectionist will say, "That's not 100%. That's like nothing! Incomplete! It's not all there!" But think about it for a second.

You still have 3/4 of a dinner made. Obviously there *is* progress. It's not black or white. If you stick with a goal 75% of the time, *it's okay*. You still did most of it – in other words, you're still much closer to the goal than you were before. Fight the inner urge to think that if you weren't 6/7 days adherent to your game plan, you won't see progress. Even 2/7 days with better habits than you had previously *will give you permanent results for life.*

***

Here's the bottom line. Perfectionism and beating yourself up is not useful in achieving your goals. Beyond making us constantly feel like crap, that nothing we ever do is good enough, it actually makes it *harder* to achieve our health goals. Sometimes the bar is just set too high. Sometimes nothing we ever do is good enough. Sometimes we see progress, but it's not *good* enough progress or not *fast* enough. And sometimes it's just *slow progress* that leaves us incredibly discouraged after a week of not seeing any results. But there's one final big problem here. Remember how I mentioned *The Key* early on in this book? It's made up of *The Narrative* (our psychology), + tiny daily habits?

The narrative is that (usually negative) voice in our head. The more we reinforce this perfectionist part of ourselves, the harder we get on ourselves, and the louder the narrative becomes.

"I told you that you always fail. You always set these stupid, huge goals and never reach them."

"What's the point in trying? You always fail anyway."

"You don't deserve setting aside time for yourself. You have a busy career and family you need to take care of, stop being so selfish and investing time and money into yourself."

"I'm going to be like this for life. My mom was like this, and most of my siblings are... it's not worth trying."

"I give up. Nothing works (or works fast enough), so I might as well just eat the foods I love and enjoy life."

"You deserve this, it's just once, and you still have the rest of the week to clean up your act. You worked so hard today anyway."

The more we support the inner perfectionist, the more we procrastinate, strengthen the negative narrative, beat ourselves up, the more we prevent the most important thing of all: progress. We're going to go deep into *The Narrative* in part two of the book, and how to conquer it. But for now, we need to conquer another horseman: the myth of the perfect time.

Chapter Recap: I Came, I Saw, I Failed.

☐ **Perfectionism.** Perfectionism (being rigid, beating ourselves up, thinking it's black or white, etc.) is not a useful mindset for being successful.

☐ **Black and white thinking.** Things are rarely black or white. Goal setting tends to make us think, "I'm either there, or I'm not yet" which clearly isn't true. The more we think of things as black and white the more we introduce stress and anxiety to the goal process.

☐ **Emphasize progress – not the end goal.** Overemphasis on the end goal "Losing 20 pounds" just leads to anxiety. Every day we think about how far away we are. The way to stay focused is instead to focus on today – did I do the habits I said I would to get one step closer? Track daily habits, instead of just daily progress or what the scale says.

☐ **Don't beat yourself up over getting derailed.** Rather than falling into periods of self-guilt, self-pity and self-hatred, just remember that the sooner we begin, the sooner we arrive. The health we want is on the other side of a couple habits, repeated a couple thousand times. Just get back on track and begin again with habit #1.

When The Planets Align,
I'm Going to Look and Feel
Like a Million Bucks!
(The Myth of the Perfect Time)

"It had long since come to my attention that people of accomplishment rarely sat back and let things happen to them. They went out and happened to things."

– LEONARDO DA VINCI

Just the other day I was overhearing a conversation between two people in a busy coffee shop: *"These past few years have been really, really tough for me, nothing has been working out and lining up – and now with mercury in retrograde I've been feeling really off. It just hasn't been the right time for my life to line up. But thankfully my chart is looking better now – this year is looking amazing so I guess it's time to start!"*

Now, regardless of whether or not you believe in astrology, that's not the point – the point is that this person genuinely believed that there was a perfect time to begin building her life, and take control of her health. But there's something scary beneath this: almost every successful, healthy person I've ever met told me the same thing: there is no "right time," that things usually only get harder as we get older, and that today is the best day to start anything – because most things are a process and take *time*. At the end of the day, those of us who wait, thinking there's a "right time" are missing one huge principle that most successful people get.

Why The "Right Time" Never Comes

Here's a thing about life that I've observed – we're typically one of two people: The first kind is someone who takes responsibility for our life, and acknowledges that almost everything about our current life is the way it is because of choices we've made. The second is someone who blames the world, forces outside them, or their circumstances for the way their life is. The first person's life is filled with feelings of personal responsibility, and the latter, blame. But there's another big thing.

People that tend to wait, and wait for "ideal timing" fail to understand what success really looks like and how to get there. They don't understand that it's a process, and instead are obsessed with the event – that one, magic, crystalizing moment when we're "there." Here's what that really looks like.

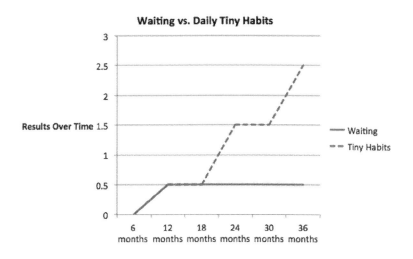

Consider this: many of us that wait for "the right time" fail to understand what success really looks like, and how we can get there. Let's say losing 20 pounds takes 1000 repetitions of a tiny habit like cooking dinner at home. We have to repeat it a certain amount of times for maximal benefits, and in order to do it 1000 times takes a certain period of time that is difficult to speed up. If it really took us 1,000 repetitions of a tiny habit, starting sooner is better than starting later, right?

If we start today, we can clock out 300+ days by the end of the year, before our friend who is waiting for some day over the rainbow when they're magically working less. That's potentially a couple thousand repetitions of some key habits. Take a look at the picture above. Initially, the first six months are almost identical. Let's just say you and your friend start at the same time.

But rather than starting off by going to the gym four hours a day like your friend does (and doing some crash diet that involves only grapefruits), you decide you're going to track very simple habits each day. Your friend quickly elapses your progress and leaves you in the dust – they reach that initial weight loss quicker than you.

But inevitably what happens?

Once the going gets tough (usually 4-8 weeks in), and they plateau or need to do something different, they usually push harder and do more, and then quit. But you're on a different timeline. You know that consistent, daily habits will get you to where you want to be, it's just a matter of adding the powerful multiplier: time. So even though your progress might've been slower than your friend, zoom out and look at the *entire year now*, or even the next few years.

Month 12 - a *year* into taking little, regular action appears to make little difference between the group taking barely any action, and just waiting for things to happen – but what you can't tell is that they're on a flat line, or downward curve. It's just so subtle and so minute that you don't realize it until years later. That's how "the weight creeps up" as we get older. It isn't until a year and a half in (month #18) do we really see the habit group take off, in an almost exponential growth pattern.

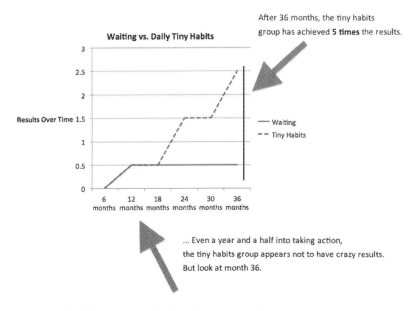

After 36 months, the tiny habits group has achieved **5 times** the results.

... Even a year and a half into taking action, the tiny habits group appears not to have crazy results. But look at month 36.

And then finally, at month 36, three *years* into repeating this simple, daily habit for thousands of repetitions, the tiny habit group is 5 times more successful than the group waiting for the proper timing. So they've lost 5x the amount of weight. That's 5 pounds versus 25 pounds. They've saved 5x the money. That's investing $50,000 instead of $10,000. And they've accomplished 5x as many goals. They've excelled at a new hobby, reversed diabetes, taken up a brand new career, and transformed their life. And it was all because they understood the very simple science of success.

The Critical Mindset That Changes Everything

Imagine this. Once we fully understand that health is a *process*, and not a magical event we arrive at when we have more time, money, friends, and when our kids are at college – we realize this big truth: Health is just a million tiny things, done over time, and there is no better time than right now – regardless of the alignment of the planets or the stars. We still have to start *some* day, and we still have to take 1,000 actions along the path. Once we change our approach, we quickly realize that we can achieve literally anything we've daydreamed about. Life opens up and seems much more like a playground, because we realize that the sooner we start something, the sooner we arrive.

Like everything I talk about here, the power of tiny habits, and the power of psychology are simply amazing in their ability to transform your entire life once you grasp them. Three things in particular, unrelated to health, will also improve once you grasp these.

Every goal in life will seem attainable – with time.

Once you understand this huge mindset shift, all goals seem attainable – with time – no matter how impossible they seem now. When we see an Olympian performing, it seems superhuman, and to most of us, Olympians *are* superhuman. But you only see them at their peak, their five minutes of fame. You don't see ten years training six hours a day, seven days a week. When you realize that getting your dream body, losing 30 pounds, boosting your energy, or reversing a chronic health condition is like planting an apple tree – it begins to make sense.

You plant a seed today. You water it for 30 days. Now you have a sapling. You water it for 300 days, now you have a shrub. You want it for 3,000 days, now you have a tree with beautiful, delicious apples. This is how achieving anything works. The sooner you plant the seed, the sooner you get the life you want.

You'll become richer and happier.

"Whoaaa Alex, you're becoming a financial coach now? Nope! Here's the thing: happiness and yes, wealth, also follow *this exact same rule!* It's that whole, save $2 a day for 30 years thing. Water the seed every day of your bank account, and you accumulate huge wealth. Or, better yet, you start building a side business just one or two hours a day after work, and three years later you get to quit your job and do what you love, having replaced your day job income. The sooner you sow that first seed, the sooner you arrive.

We'll shift from blaming others for our lack of success, health or happiness, to taking full responsibility for our life.

This is perhaps the best of all. What would every day be like if you *knew* you were in control? I mean imagine that – you could change *anything* you wanted – your job, your financial status, your health, where you lived, how you lived, your happiness – anything. Most of us don't believe these things are possible, but they are. When you finally commit to being responsible for everything in your life, you feel in control. You are empowered – which literally means you have the power. You decide that yes, there are some things you can't change, but there's a lot you can.

Most of it we can change. Imagine what it'd feel like to wake up every day and realize we can live *any* life we want, have any health we want, and have any level of financial success we want? Powerful, right? Once we ditch the idea that there's a "right time" to begin, we'll begin the most important psychological shift we could ever make: taking consistent, tiny, daily action.

> "The best time to plant a tree was 20 years ago. The next best time is today."
>
> - Chinese Proverb

***

Everyone is looking for the *one* thing. And that's why nobody finds it. It's because it isn't *one* thing, and is instead *a thousand things*. So that's why so many of us get the frustrating "I'm not quite sure what the biggest thing was" when we ask someone who transformed their health for their best advice. It's because there *wasn't just one thing*. There were thousands.

It was the eating strategies, eating a bit more of this, a bit less of that. It was walking 10 minutes a day. It was a bit of stress management. It was a bit more sleep. It was becoming a bit happier. It was drinking a bit more water and a bit less coffee. And these thousand things created a synergy of effects. It's like changing your nutrition. It's easily the biggest thing you can do to transform how you look and feel (it's 80% of the work in a transformation). But if you throw in exercise, now you have another multiplier.

If you sleep more, there's another one. If you meditate a half hour a day, now you've got another huge multiplier. The synergy caused by all of these little, daily things is bigger than their own individual effects.

Losing The Frustrating Last 10 Pounds

Let me share with you how losing those last ten pounds goes – in real life – not in celebrity magazines or movies. The last ten pounds can be frustrating to lose because your body is already close to a normalized weight, and thus it's more reluctant to let go of weight. Near the extremes, losing weight or feeling a lot better is much easier, and even small changes produce big results (like my 400 pound CPR instructor I mentioned earlier). But the last ten can be tough. Let me tell you what the real silver bullet looks like in practice.

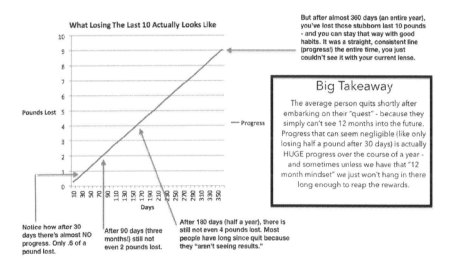

So what's going on here? This is a great example of the "100 day rule." So much of the time, we quit right before we've struck gold. We often excitedly embark on a new health regime or new meditation regime or new yoga routine, and if we aren't magically most of the way to our goals within 30 days, we quit. "I just wasn't seeing results and got discouraged. I wonder if I was even given good advice in the first place." Take a look at the picture above. This is a *realistic* (i.e. real) look at how a person loses their last 10 pounds to get into crazy cover-of-the-magazine shape. So let's take a look at some benchmarks, looking *purely* at weight loss.

Month 1 – First 30 days.

Not even one pound lost. That's around .6 of a pound. Here's what that looks like in reality. You step on the scale one day, you see a pound lost (wahoo!), and then a week later, the weight is back to normal (ugh). Negligible. Not noticeable at all.

Month 2 – First 60 days.

Around 1.3 pounds lost. That's almost nothing, once again. You can drink too much water in a day, and "gain" 1.3 pounds. You can run around on a hot summer day and lose 3-5 pounds of water weight. 1.3 is usually not noticeable.

Month 3 – First 90 days.

Notice how it's now ¼ *of a year*. A large chunk of the *year* has gone by, and you've only lost 1.3 pounds. By far the majority of people quit here, because results "aren't happening," but since you read this book you how it works and keep going. You know that real results happen over time – with commitment to daily habits that don't seem that miraculous. After 90 days, you've only lost two pounds. *Two* pounds! Absolute insanity. You must be crazy. Why bother even continuing? All these daily habits you're doing, and 90 days later you still haven't lost any noticeable weight.

Month 6 – First 180 days.

You're right around four pounds lost. Really not that impressive, but *finally* you are seeing results on the scale, your pants are a bit looser, and things are feeling different – much different. You notice a flatter belly, there's less bulge in your clothes, and you're noticing a difference in the mirror. The muffin top or gut is disappearing little by little. But it took *half a year* to see any noticeable results. 99% of people have already quit.

Month 9 – First 270 days.

You now lost around six and a half pounds – now it's getting noticeable. It seems like it's happening quickly now, almost like each time you look in the mirror, less of your stomach exists, and more of the toned, defined lines you've always wanted have started to show.

Month 12 – First 360 days.

Wahoo! The final 10 pounds lost. Your stomach looks toned and fit, or if you're a man, you've finally got that six-pack starting to show that you've been dreaming about and observing in the movies. It's a reality. Friends approach you – "Wow! You look amazing; you're an overnight success! How did you do it so quickly?"

Uhh.

Quickly? What do you mean? "It seems like I just saw you last year and you had a noticeable "pooch" and now you have an incredibly beach body." What they didn't see, what they *never* see, were the thousands of tiny daily actions that you took to get to where you are today. In fact, that's what most of us *never* see – no one said it had to be hard work, but you *do* have to do the work, you do have to do those daily habits.

They didn't see this: Ten minutes a day of walking, which amounted to: 3,650 minutes (around 61 hours) on the road walking around your town. Four home cooked meals a week, which amounted to: 208 home made meals cooked. Fifteen minutes of yoga a day, 4x a week, which amounted to: 3,120 minutes (52 hours) on the floor of a yoga studio bending and sweating. There were the three tiny habits, per day, seven days a week. Which was 7,665 habits that you actively, consciously practiced to get to where you are today.

Yeah, sure. An *overnight success*. *This* is what most people won't show you. *This* is the most 'secret' of all the secrets out there. The missing link that virtually guarantees success no matter what diet you engage in, no matter what change you're trying to make in your life, no matter where you are now or what kind of person you are now. No matter how far away, you can make it a reality. You just need to understand *The Key*.

Chapter Recap: The Myth of The Perfect Time

☐ **There is no perfect time to start.** Waiting for the perfect time implies that there is magically going to be a moment where everything is perfect in life, you have more time, more energy, more happiness, and more willpower. But the moment rarely arrives if we wait for it.

☐ **The right time never comes.** The longer we wait, the longer we get frustrated, all because we realize that this is a big myth. We also tend to assume that health transformation takes a lot of time each day – which isn't necessarily true. It just takes consistency.

☐ **Begin before you are ready.** Does walking ten minutes a day really take that much time to get started? Is it dramatically inconveniencing you? The good news is that by doing this, it'll snowball, and will naturally lead to other tiny habits that improve your life.

PART 2

The Solution: The Raw Truth About Little Things That Produce Massive Results (Without Hours In The Gym)

Why We Fail
(And What To Do About It)

There's a secret that the most successful, healthy, vital people know that most people don't. It's not actually *what* we're doing that's the most important part of being successful or healthy (even though it's important). It's just a matter of doing it. To be more specific, it's about creating *systems* in your own life to go from meditating just once, to meditating every day. It's about going from eating healthy on Mondays, to eating healthy most days of the week.

If we don't do what we said we would – figuring out *why* we didn't. In the following chapters, I'm going to introduce you to a few principles, daily habits, and systems that you can apply *right now* after you read each chapter. The first thing I'm going to introduce you to is the "systems philosophy," which is a fundamentally different success philosophy that bypasses thinking about the "eating less, moving more" advice as the reason for failure. It's all about changing our *behavior*. Nothing changes in our life until the fundamental choices we make each moment are different.

Next, I'm going to introduce you my short, million dollar daily ritual. Yes, it's worth that and much more. The point of the daily ritual is that it gives you a daily *system* for staying focused, motivated, and clear on what needs to happen today in order to get to where we want to be. And most of all, it'll help us do this without using massive willpower, discipline, effort or some limitless channel of motivation. After that I'm going to show you how to get over *The Narrative* that may be sabotaging you. It'll help you silence the inner voice, so you can take action every day without being harassed by a brain that tells you "You're a failure" or "you're not worth it" or "why bother trying?"

Remember – the mind is half the game. It sounds a bit strange and esoteric, but I'll give you *plenty* of examples of people that overcame *The Narrative*, and how it dramatically improved their life beyond just their health and weight. Finally, I'm going to show you several daily habits for actually applying this in your life, today. From there, I'll show you how to stay focused and maintain these changes on the road ahead, and what key traits separate success from failure at the end of the day.

The Power of Sticky Notes: The World's Most Sophisticated Life Transformation System (The Systems Philosophy)

So how do you, you know, actually *do it?* How do you take yourself from thinking about eating more vegetables, walking more, going to yoga more, meditating regularly, de-cluttering your life, sleeping better, and stressing less to actually doing it? It's all from a fundamentally different approach: thinking in terms of systems in our life that are causing us to fail.

Think about it: everything in nature follows a system. In temperate climates, spring, summer, fall, and winter always follow each other. They just do. It's a law of nature. It's a system. It's repeatable, predictable, and 100% guaranteed. It's something we can predict, and thus rely on. Think about the best companies in the world: everything they do is systematized. Coffee shop employees are trained regarding what they should say, how to present the coffee, systems for making the coffee the same way every day, systems for grabbing the tea bag without using their fingers, systems for handling lines, systems for handling grumpy customers, and so on.

All this results in *predictable, regular results* the company can depend on. This is critical to the company working effectively and being successful at what they do. Most importantly, *when something goes wrong*, they know exactly where to look in order to fix it. When something isn't working, it's never a big confusing question about why it didn't work or who the bad employee was. They just look at the checklist process and see what didn't work and why. But what you may not realize is that your own daily habits are systems too. There are usually repeated triggers that set off bad habits and put them into motion.

Here are a few examples of what I mean.

System #1: Habitual overeating, getting fast food, and stress eating.

I told you about Mike earlier in the book, who recently got a brand new job and was working hard to prove his worth. He was working twelve hours a day, and at the end of the day, because of the stress and anxiety he would go to the same Chinese takeout place and get the same two bottles of his favorite beer, plop down on the couch at home, and go into a coma for a while.

He told me that this was pretty much *required* for him to function after work – otherwise he would be snappy with his wife and his kids. So think about it. This is a predictable routine. We know that:

A. Stress is Mike's trigger
B. Pretty much any day where Mike works 12+ hours a day, he's stressed
C. When Mike is stressed he craves Chinese food and beer to decompress
D. Mike feels better after he indulges

In fact, this system works like clockwork for him. Twelve hour days + stress = Cravings.

System #2: Work stress.

Sandra is an ambitious young woman based in New York City working at a local startup. She loves the startup space with the passion, the people, the fire, the rush and the variety of projects she gets to work on. The only problem is that she's basically the person right under the CEO, so she's the one who gets most of the flack when something doesn't go right. With 30+ people to manage and make sure everything runs smoothly, she's the direct link from the CEO to the worker bees.

Recently, Sandra got into a huge argument with the CEO because he expected her to run a successful marketing campaign by herself, when she was understaffed and underfunded. He blew up in her face (which embarrassed her), so she walked out. She took a minute to leave the office, walk around the block a few times, take some deep breaths, and then go back in. As she sat texting her friend on her phone, a man next to her was smoking a cigarette and said, "You look like you could use one." She never smoked before, but she figured, "yeah, I sure could." She took a deep breath, and it was instant relief.

The rest was history – any time she and the CEO got into it together, her ritual became the "let's get some fresh air" ritual, which she associated with the deep relief she got from a cigarette. This habit then generalized to any time she felt stress from any source in her life. The cigarette was her best friend. For Sandra, it was job stress + walking outside to decompress = smoke a cigarette. Any time those two conditions were present the third was too.

System #3: The coffee trigger.

Just the other day, in my part of town it was your quintessential gloomy Monday. Getting out of bed? Ugh. Showing up at the office? Ugh. Trying to be in a remotely good mood? Ugh. Attempting to accomplish a bit of work? Ugh. About an hour into my workday, I realized I hadn't done anything yet, so I got up to take a quick break. As I walked around, I smelled coffee coming from the coffee shop around the corner, so I decided to walk over.

I got a nice dark roast, quickly walked back to the office, sat down and worked for three hours straight. Even though I didn't get any caffeine high, it was like I was struck with the magical elixir of productivity. Interestingly, over the next few months, not only did I go from being a non-coffee drinker to a coffee drinker, I also started drinking coffee multiple times per day, any time I wanted to do work. Coffee had successfully become my trigger for work, and any time I wasn't productive, all it took was the smell and the first sip of a coffee, and I was in the zone. For me the system became coffee + work = productive.

So, systems follow predictable routines. Imagine if all of your *positive* health and weight loss habits were pretty much automatic?

Imagine if rather than thinking about meditating or just doing it once a week, you did it every day like you've really wanted to? Imagine if you saw the wrong foods, and didn't go anywhere near them? Imagine if you had a craving, but then had a system you could count on for not caving to the hunger? Imagine if you had special bulk cooking methods each Sunday night so that even if you were exhausted during the week, you came home to a full fridge with a delicious meal you just had to heat up? Imagine if any time you found yourself feeling discouraged yet again, you had motivational systems lined up, and a few minutes later, you were *on fire,* ready to roll and make it happen again?

***

Let's be honest, we all have some habits or repeated behaviors in our lives that clearly just aren't doing it for us. That afternoon or late night sugar habit? It probably needs some fixing. Or what about those couple beers or glasses of wine we drink when we're out with the guys or the girls a couple times a week? Or maybe it's just the "I think I'll make an entire box of brownies and destroy it by myself" habit.

Listen, we all have these, it's human! But the ultimate question isn't what we're doing; it's why we're doing it. Let's take cravings for example. Many people know why they have cravings, and what causes them. But from working with people, I know that an equal number also have no clue what causes their cravings or what to do about it. So the most important part for these people is having *awareness* of what triggers it (if it's emotional). In fact, we can use the food cravings, smoking, and the coffee-trigger in the same vein.

Something triggers all three of these situations, and if we don't know what causes them, we have no idea how to regain control over them. A really basic psychological tool I use involves the power of the sticky note. You can use a piece of paper, your phone, a notepad, or any other note-taking device.

Here's all you need to do. Any time you have one of these "episodes" like you find yourself smoking, having a craving or drinking that fifth cup of coffee, you write down two things. First, what you were just doing before it happened? Second, what you were just thinking, feeling or experiencing? Here's what you'll discover. You may find that you have cravings every single day at three pm because you're working on the same boring work project every single day this time, and it's your way of "taking a break." What were you just doing? Working on the spreadsheet for the asset allocation project (yawn). What were you just feeling? Bored. What did you learn? When you're bored, you tend to crave food.

You may find that any time you feel overwhelmed at work and you really just need to "get away," you begin craving the feeling of getting some fresh air and smoking a cigarette. The cigarette has become your best buddy for stress relief. What were you just doing? Arguing with your manager over a new project and the short deadline. What were you just feeling? Stressed beyond belief, and frustrated. What did you learn? When you're stressed, the cigarette cravings hit. And you may find that, like for me, coffee has become your work trigger. You drank coffee for so many years first thing in the morning that the association of coffee + work = productivity. And now you have a hard time being productive without your coffee, even if the caffeine content is negligible.

What were you just doing? Working on the first project of the morning on Monday. What were you just feeling? Unproductive. What did you learn? When you feel unproductive, coffee helps you become more productive. So this sticky note exercise is an extremely simple but sophisticated exercise for figuring out why we do what we do, as far as bad habits go. Here's why I bring up all this "systems and habits" stuff, and why it's a fundamentally different approach: when you "fail" temporarily – it's never you, it's the *system* you set up which became habits and behaviors.

Let me say that again. When something doesn't go the way we planned with our health, instead of saying "what did I do wrong?" ask yourself "what system, habit, or series of events led up to this?" So rather than blaming ourselves and yet again being disappointed and feeling guilty, when we get that it's really about *behaviors* not working – we know exactly where to go to improve – our habits and the systems underlying them. This entire process serves one purpose only: insight.

Unless we have insight into the inner workings of our life and our mind, we just run on autopilot. We continue to complain about the things we usually do. We go through the same routine that makes us unhappy. And we eat the same things and engage in the same behaviors even though they lead us down a road we don't want to go down. Insight and awareness are the first step to overcoming the bad habits in our life. Remember, rather than thinking about what happened, ask yourself why it did, and what system led up to it. Rather than saying "I was stress eating again" ask yourself, "What system, habits, and series of events led up to this?"

In the coming chapters, we're going to walk through how to anchor in good new habits to turn them into regular, predictable systems, using the power of the *master the day* habit, daily rituals, routines, and more. The most important chapters here are the first two: The narrative, and *Master The* Day - the million dollar daily ritual.

Chapter Recap: The Power of Post-it Notes - The Systems Philosophy

☐ **When you can't stick to a habit (or have a bad habit) think in terms of systems.** What is it about your routine that is causing you to keep engaging in this negative behavior over and over? If you keep finding yourself drinking six cups of coffee a day, why is that? The easiest way is using a sticky note, your phone, a notepad, or something else and just tracking the behavior. For anything repetitive and damaging write down: What did I do, and why did I do it? What was I doing just before it?

☐ **Insight as to why habits and systems occur is the most important part of changing our behavior.** Once you use the sticky note method you can figure out what's going on. Okay, I drink six cups of coffee a day because I associate coffee with work – even if it doesn't give me any more energy. Now you have awareness around why it happens, which disables the autopilot lifestyle (AL).

My Momma Said I'm a Lazy Good-For-Nothin'... (Overcoming The Story Inside Your Head)

Overwhelmingly, despite what "experts" say, health and weight loss isn't just about eating less and moving more: it's about understanding our own mind. Check out a few of these stories readers have shared with me:

"I have pretty much given up since I have always failed... it has made me afraid of failure so I have learned to stop trying."

> "Hello, Mr. Heyne. I am struggling with my own fear of failure. I don't usually diet because I have pretty much given up since I have always failed. I have always been fat, at least from the age of 6. My grandmother would use weight loss as a methods of abuse. I won't go into that sordid history, but it has made me afraid of failure so I have learned to stop trying. However, I have dealt with depression for years and I'm sick of it all. At this point, it's either change or die."

"Nothing will change, you're always going to be like that..."

"I want to lose weight to wear my old clothes and not have fat hanging out from places. For my height I need to be leaner. Everyone on my husband's family is lean and thin and I can feel the judgment in their eyes (and sometimes it comes in their words too) that I must be eating something wrong or just being lazy (or inherit it a.k.a blaming my parents) or it is my mistake that I am fat. My attempts to not eat fried food is ridiculed as 'nothing will change, you will remain as you are'...it haunts me and has become a personal battle for me now."

"I deserve food at the end of a long day as a reward."

"Ok...I get up at 6am and leave the house at 7:15. I don't have breakfast as I can't stomach it. I might have a breakfast bar at 10:30. Between 1 and 1:30pm is lunch - I tend to have a sandwich or a cup of soup. By the time I get home at 6pm I am ravenous and stuff high calorie, high sugar food into me. I usually make a pasta meal and I have a portion that is too big. I buy fruit and veggies but don't eat them. I don't plan well as have got into a rut of eating rubbish and tend to buy the same stuff each week with no real idea of what to have. On a good (planned) week I'll have spaghetti bolognaise; chicken korma; venison burger; pasta bake, that kind of thing. Lunches are difficult, as I have no idea what to make. I also eat cake, chocolate, ice cream after a bad day or when I'm tired or if I feel I deserve some TLC...all the while I know I am damaging myself."

You know what I find interesting here? Overwhelmingly, these three readers didn't mention much about their diet. They talked about what's going on *in their mind*. They're talking about the story going on – *The Narrative* – whether it's the story they have told themselves, or a story that their mother, partner, boss, or friend told them. It's the story that most often damages us and holds us back, and it's re-writing the inner story that most often gets us back on track.

Like I said, this is a bit "out there" for the average person – everyone just wants to address the symptoms of poor health and weight gain, but no one wants to treat the underlying cause. The underlying cause of repetitive failure is often a story. Remember *The Key?* The two fundamentally different approaches I noticed over and over in the success stories were two simple but important things: *"The Narrative"* + Little Daily Habits. So what on earth is the narrative, and how is it the #1 thing preventing me from getting to where I want to be? Shouldn't I just be eating less and moving more?

Hardly.

Here's what I mean. The Narrative (with a capital "T") is *the* story. You know, the big, main story behind our lives. It's the meaning we give to the events around us. We all have repetitive problems in our lives. Sometimes we feel as though the entire world is conspiring against us – the economy is garbage, and thus we can't get a job or can't get a raise. My parents were overweight, diabetic, and had cancer, and thus I'm probably toast – there's not much I can do to change. In this case, the narrative is *blame*.

Sometimes it's just a story of continual *failure*. You read the story above of the reader who had failed so many times in his life, that he wondered why he should even bother trying again. "Might as well just eat what tastes good and enjoy life!" You can imagine how this might carry over to other aspects of his life – his relationships, his personal dreams, passions and aspirations. The underlying story that keeps playing out is this: "Everything I try to do, I fail at." So what keeps showing up in this person's life? Failure. He sees failure at virtually everything he tries.

Sometimes the narrative is even more serious like: "I hate myself." A long time ago, a female friend of mine was dating a guy that she was really interested in. *"Finally* I found a guy that likes me too! This is going to be amazing." So over time she got closer and closer to him, and eventually they were getting pretty serious, and the strangest thing happened: She very clearly was sabotaging the relationship. She was so uncomfortable with being loved, with being herself, with being someone that a man was *actually interested in* ("for once in her life"), that she started acting hostile, squeamish and weird.

She suddenly got so insecure that "he couldn't possibly love her" that she started avoiding his dinner requests since she figured he was just going to leave her for another girl anyway. She pulled away prematurely, because she figured it was going to end at some point, and can you imagine what happened to the guy?

He was wondering the entire time what he did wrong. And sure enough, over the months of her withdrawing and randomly acting bizarre, he did pull away for good. Ironically, the process of her pulling away to protect herself caused him to do the same. In this case, the story is *"No one could possibly love me,"* and sure enough, it shows up over and over again. The narrative just reinforces itself over and over, unless we address it, confront it, and question it.

"I'm just too lazy and unmotivated."

We often say things like "ugh, I'm so lazy" when it comes time for things like exercising or eating more of the right foods (or cooking). Regardless of whether or not you really *are* lazy, just take a look at how this narrative might affect your daily decisions in a few scenarios. Imagine you're trying to apply for a brand new dream job you discovered. The interviewer sends you a *long* interview form, about three pages to fill out, plus a personal cover letter, and some references. It's longer than you've ever seen one before.

"This job looks amazing but... ugh, it looks like a lot of work." Do you fill it out right away and apply sooner to get noticed, or delay? If we have an, "I'm just a lazy person" narrative, it's pretty obvious which option we'll pick, which directly sabotages us. Here's another example. You're presented with a rare, once in a lifetime opportunity to pursue something you're passionate about: Let's say it's marine biology. You'll get to go to Fiji for a summer and study the local fish species, giant clams, sharks, and more. It's what you've wanted to do your entire life.

Plus, there's something more: A famous National Geographic photographer will be there with some other well known scientists in the field that could secure you an incredible job after. There's one catch: In order to afford it, since you have to pay for the $2,000 flight, it means you're going to have to work an extra four hours every day, including weekends, for the next *six months* to pay for it. You'll need a second job. Let's say you're working fulltime, 9-5. That means you'll get home, and have to work 6-10, Monday through Friday, and then also on your Saturday and Sunday. "I'm lazy and unmotivated." This is a dream job and once in a lifetime opportunity, do you do the work and take it?

It's clear what option the person with the "I'm lazy" narrative will pick. It's amazing how many things we write out of our lives (without ever giving them a chance to even become a reality) because of the story we tell ourselves. Here's one final narrative. "I'm so unlucky, nothing ever works out for me." Alex wakes up in the morning, hops out of bed, and falls over hitting his face on the door in front of him. "Ugh, Monday mornings." It's no big deal and he continues getting ready. As he's standing in line at the local coffee shop, the barista spills the scalding hot coffee on his wrist, *and* overcharges him. Still – it's not a big deal.

On his way out of the coffee shop, a pigeon poops on his head. "Just my luck." Some weeks later, his girlfriend dumps him for another guy – one of his friends. A recent job promotion he was planning on getting overlooked him – and they picked a new rookie to get it. He gets fired. As the months go by he doesn't even apply for jobs, "I'm unlucky so I won't get any of these anyway." He doesn't. And more and more he falls into this negative spiral of hating life, hating everyone, and hating himself: "*Nothing* ever works out, this life is such a scam, such BS, why do I even go on?" And you know what's interesting? This is a repetitive pattern in his life.

Before this life phase, he always described himself as an "unlucky" person – where good things seemed to happen to everyone else, everyone except for him. Sure enough, just like he describes himself, he appears to be an objectively unlucky person. What's going on with Alex? Could he really be that unlucky? Here's what's incredibly powerful about these narratives: *none of them are actually 100% true.* Well, they begin as truth. They are shadows of the truth. Sometimes they *are* true, or have been true to a certain extent.

We really might have failed the past few times we tried to diet. Our mom really might have told us that we're "doomed to be this way" or we're "so dumb sometimes." Usually, they begin as truth, or half-truths. But the problem is that they turn into a full-blown story that we keep for the rest of our lives – subconsciously sabotaging ourselves as we reinforce this belief that we can't do something or that we're a certain way. They're just stories we tell ourselves. That's why I call it *The Narrative*. We often have one (or a few) predominant stories going on in our head.

Consider the luck example, since it seems to be an extremely common superstition. In the early 2000s a study was done by Richard Wiseman to see if whether people *believed* they were lucky influenced how lucky they objectively were.[11] Here's how it went:

"I placed advertisements in national newspapers and magazines, asking for people who considered themselves exceptionally lucky or unlucky to contact me. Over the years, 400 extraordinary men and women have volunteered to participate in my research; the youngest eighteen, a student, the oldest eighty-four, a retired accountant. They were drawn from all walks of life – businessmen, factory workers, teachers, housewives, doctors, secretaries, and salespeople. All were kind enough to let me put their lives and minds under the microscope. Take the case of chance opportunities. Lucky people consistently encounter such opportunities whereas unlucky people do not. I carried out a very simple experiment to discover whether this was due to differences in their ability to spot such opportunities. I gave both lucky and unlucky people a newspaper, and asked them to look through it and tell me how many photographs were inside.

On average, the unlucky people took about two minutes to count the photographs whereas the lucky people took just seconds. Why? Because the second page of the newspaper contained the message "Stop counting – There are 43 photographs in this newspaper." This message took up half of the page and was written in type that was over two inches high. It was staring everyone straight in the face, but the unlucky people tended to miss it and the lucky people tended to spot it. Just for fun, I placed a second large message half way through the newspaper. This one announced: "Stop counting, tell the experimenter you have seen this and win $250." Again, the unlucky people missed the opportunity because they were still too busy looking for photographs."

Incredible, huh? Just based on whether or not these people *described* themselves as lucky or unlucky, *actually made them lucky or unlucky.* The lucky people actually were more likely to use their intuition, see and seize rare opportunities, were more open and positive and thus noticed more things, and overall were more "lucky." They literally were luckier. So if just *thinking* you're lucky makes you luckier, imagine the narrative you have currently going on and how it might be affecting your life?

Can you imagine the kinds of outcomes we generate in our own lives – and in our own health – when we tell ourselves that we're a certain way? What about saying that we can't do a certain thing? *"I can't lose weight, my mother was always overweight."* What about saying that we always do a certain thing, like fail?

"What's the point? Everything I've tried has never worked in the long run." For example, you tell yourself you'll never be slim, but that can be a lie – something your mom told you because she was envious of your thin, youthful body that she never could regain. This might sound sick, like a deranged story you might see on a reality TV show, but I can assure you I've heard plenty of them. Sometimes a person comes from a poor or immigrant family where it's shameful to leave food on the plate, because the elder generations went through extreme hardship trying to survive and feed their families. As a person ages, they continue to have this "clean the plate, no matter what's put in front of you" mentality, which can cause problems.

The most important thing we need to understand first is this: the narrative is a lie. It may be based on truth, but repeating this story in your head just prevents you from succeeding in the future. The easiest way to begin tracking the narrative in your head is simple: take out a notepad or use a note program on your phone, and simply *write down every thought in your head for a week*. Sounds crazy, and it sounds like a lot of work, but trust the process. Track the story in your head based on whatever aspect of your life you want improving – if it's the relationship with food or exercise, write down your thoughts or words when you talk about these things.

How are you describing eating healthy? Going for walks? Reading health books? Cooking at home? Those usually reflect your reality. Maybe you keep describing eating healthy as exhausting because of the "boring, bland tasting food." Maybe you keep telling yourself that being healthy "is really time consuming, and I just can't squeeze it into my schedule." You might be really surprised at what comes up. You might realize that the association between what we think about, and what our reality looks like, is *uncanny*. It's insanely accurate.

Here's how to silence the narrative and replace it with a better one that inspires you and keeps you focused.

Imagine the Narrative As a Totally Separate Person

So now you know *what* the narrative is, what it's saying, and you realize that the narrative is often a lie or a repetitive story you tell yourself which sabotages you and prevents success, let's talk about conquering it. The problem is that we often identify with the lie over time, as the narrative repeats itself and occupies mental space. So after all this work, after understanding what the narrative is and how it negatively affects your life, let's talk about shutting it up for good. I could suggest all kinds of things that would make the narrative quieter, like meditation, but I know you're busy and probably won't do them. (Notice the narrative there?)

Here's a little exercise you can practice. Imagine the narrative as a totally separate person. So let's say one of those repetitive voices pops up: "You always fail at dieting when you try each year, so why bother trying again?"

"I'm so unlucky, *nothing* ever works out for me."

"Wow... I look awful."

Immediately imagine it as *a different person*. You can even give it a name to really emphasize that it's something separate from you. The meditative traditions like to call it the "monkey mind" but if you give it an actual name, it's much easier to imagine it as a separate part of you that's trying to sabotage you. Let's say you give the narrative the name "Annoying Nancy" or "Stupid Stan" – bonus points if it's a childhood arch nemesis that you hated. She goes off, "You're so dumb, you always do this" or "You deserve this cookie, you had a long day at work" or "You look god awful" – make sure to observe that it's not *you* saying this (and thus don't believe it), and observe that it's Annoying Nancy. "Oh it's just Annoying Nancy, she always gets loud when I start a new diet regime or read a new health book."

"Shut up Nancy, I'm busy over here."

"Stupid Stan, you're really bothering me dude. Cut the crap."

It sounds like insanity, and obviously I wouldn't have this conversation out loud, but this is a surprisingly effective way to shut up the narrative. When we take a second and pretend that it's an entirely different person – some kind of gremlin on our shoulder preventing us from getting the health, body, and life we want – it becomes easy to ignore it or shut it up.

Replace the Narrative With a Better One
(And Fill Your Mind With It)

So you know the narrative is often a lie, and is just a repetitive thought pattern. And you've given the narrative a separate name, so you realize that it's not *you* doing all this negative talking. Now we're going to figure out *why* you say it, and then give you a better narrative that actually inspires you and motivates you. So, step 1 is you understand what the narrative is, and you've realized what it's been saying. Step 2 is that you've given your narrative "voice" a new name because it's someone else. And now, step 3 is this: When your narrative goes off, ask, "Why did I say that?"

Here's an example. "You always fail at dieting, there's no point in even trying again." Why did I say that? "Well, I tried a diet in 2009, and lasted for about a week then quit. I tried a different diet in 2007 and lasted about a month, and then I just got too busy. I tried that sugar cleanse in 2006, which was just ridiculously restrictive and made me pray for death (so I gave it up). So I guess the last three diets I've tried I "failed" to keep up with. That's why I say I always fail." So do you really always fail? No, the last three fads you went on you just had a hard time sticking with. Are there possibly other things in your life that you tried and didn't fail at? Maybe you can think back to a community event where you had loads of responsibility, and you really came through for someone. Or maybe you had a personal work goal (or dream) that you did exceptionally well on. Maybe you're an awesome spouse and you consistently deliver there.

Look for other events and situations that contradict your narrative – all for the explicit purpose of showing you that *it's a lie*. It's just a voice in your head trying to sabotage you. And it's not you. Sometimes it just takes one story, and runs with it for years and decades. Sometimes it just takes the "I failed last time I tried" story, and morphs it into the "I always fail" story, which is dangerous. The sooner it gets silenced and replaced with something awesome, the sooner our life will reflect that. Keep asking, "Why did I say that?" and go deeper. Think about some of these other narratives and imagine how they might sabotage your daily life.

"I always fail, so I'm just going to fail again."

"I'm so unlucky."

"My mom said I'd always be fat, just like her."

"Money is dirty."

"It's impossible to earn a living doing something I love."

Whether it's health or just life, our minds are often filled with narratives that sabotage us. Once we spend time to actually notice the narrative, we'll realize just how insidious it is – it's everywhere, affecting every part of our life.

Replace The Narrative With Something Awesome That Inspires You

Some years back I was pretty severely depressed because nothing in my life was going how I wanted it to be. I had that classic "Oh man, how did I get here?" day. I had no job, and then a bad job. I didn't have many friends or any new hobbies, and I moved back in with my parents at the ripe old age of 24. It was pretty bad. Pretty much all day all I could think about was how much I hated my life. When I drove around town I even thought, "What's the point of any of this? All of this is so useless, this entire daily routine, the jobs, the bills – everything." My narrative became, "Everything I do throughout the day is pointless – it's all meaningless."

As you can imagine, my life very quickly became meaningless and pointless, and I fell into a deep depression. A year or two after that, when I finally started waking up from the haze, I had to really struggle to start my life over in every single aspect: my social life, my work life, my health, everything. During this time, it was a constant battle to fight the negative barrage of thoughts, because the narrative became "this is so hard, I'm never going to succeed, and it's all pointless anyway." So I gave myself a little mantra. First – I observed the narrative. I noticed that it was an overwhelmingly negative narrative. And unsurprisingly, that was the story my physical life was playing out too. I told myself that life was pointless, and sure enough, everything in my life became pointless.

Second – I pretended the narrative was a different person. Like a little demon in my head, a little devil, trying to prevent me from reaching my goals. I pretended that the narrative was the voice of resistance. Third – I replaced the narrative with a more useful one. Anytime I noticed this kind of negativity, I would replace it with a little mantra: "Smile, Deep Breath, Refocus, Do the Work." So I would start beating myself up, or *nothing* would work for a period of weeks or months, and I would start creating a bad narrative. "Oh man, you're never going to get out of this funk. Life is so pointless, this economy sucks, you're going to live with your parents until you're 40…" Then I'd repeat the little mantra to reset it. "Smile, Deep Breath, Refocus, Do the Work." I would smile and take a deep breath, and dramatically relax. I would refocus by visualizing my goal, and then "do the work" meant turn the mind off, shut up, and work on the goal.

For you, now you know the narrative, and you know how to shut it up, but then what? You replace it with something better. When the narrative has been shut up, you want to fill your mind with the vision of the future. It should be *the* vision that inspires you. I suggest a combination of things: either using an affirmation or filling it with visualizations. You've shut up the narrative, and now you repeat to yourself your goal or mantra, "I'm committed to losing 20 pounds and getting my dream body." Or you can take five seconds, and visualize yourself in the future with whatever outcome you want.

Another example: back in my depression example, when nothing in my life seemed to be working or enjoyable, with resistance all around me, after I silenced the narrative I replaced it with a vision of the future I wanted: "I'm waking up in a job I'm excited to do, working with fun, interesting people. I have dozens of close friends around me and a large network. I have a girlfriend who's adventurous and loves travel, great food, and going into New York City."

I just kept going on and on with this visualization for a minute or two when I got into a bad mood, and it really reframed that and cheered me up. And I did this a couple thousand times over the next year. In fact, that constant visualization of the "good life" I wanted, any time the narrative got loud, was one of the things that saved my life by keeping me out of that dark place that made me want to quit. But guess what's even better? Two years after that phase, *every single one* of those visualizations came true. I can't quite explain why or how, but they did.

Four months later I got my first job I didn't hate. Three months after that I fell in love for the first time ever. A year later, I had more friends than I ever had in my life. And within two years, most of the aspects of my life were "back on track" and those dark days of resistance were mostly gone 90% of the time.

The narrative reframe is powerful.

Once the narrative has been silenced, just take a few seconds to repeat an affirmation or (my favorite) just visualize the outcome you really want. The worst-case scenario is that any time you feel discouraged, this will instantly inspire you and focus you. Before we end this critical chapter on *The Narrative*, here's a quick recap of the steps.

Step #1: Pay attention to *The Narrative* throughout the day, and what it says.

Example 1: "I'm too busy to do any new kind of health regime." Example 2: "I'm afraid of looking attractive again because then I'll have no excuse for avoiding dating." The easiest way to pay attention to it is to *literally* write down the thoughts in your head for an entire week.

Step #2: Realize that the narrative is a lie.

It's another person, it's your head, and it's not you. Give the person a name. Tell it to shut up when it starts to derail you. For example: "Annoying Nancy is talking again, she's saying that I won't succeed because I always quit everything I try. Shut up Nancy."

Step #3: Ask "why" do I say this?

Example: "You're never going to be able to stick to this plan." Why did I say this? Pause for a moment and really think. "Because in 2008, 2007, and 2006, I tried different 'diets' and 'cleanses' and they were too restrictive so I didn't stick to any of them." The realization: "I don't fail all the time, I just struggled the last three times I attempted diet fads." Narrative busted. Sometimes it begins with truth, but if we tell ourselves the same story a decade later, clearly it's not that useful and only prevents progress.

Usually, any time we see a person who ends up in the same circumstances over and over (bad relationships, bad jobs, stressful financial situations, lots of anger, poor health), there's a very strong inner narrative being played out that they aren't aware of.

Step #4: Replace it with new affirmations and visualizations.

Once you've silenced the narrative, replace it with an affirmation or visualization.

Affirmation: "I'm committed to losing 20 pounds and getting my dream body. I will find a way to make the time, enjoy the process and eventually get there."

Visualization: See yourself on a vacation one year from now, not being embarrassed to walk around in your swimsuit. See yourself being *excited* to be the first person to show off. See yourself walking up stairs easily, effortlessly. See yourself springing out of bed with crazy energy. See yourself passing the cupcakes at the coffee shop with ease.

We're going to dive deep into specific visualizations, how to use them, what to visualize, and the almost *eerie* ways visualizations actually end up showing up in your life in the next chapter. One final thing: this next chapter – Habit #2 Master the Day – is the most important chapter in the book. If you don't take away *anything* from this book, just download or print out chapter two and read it a few minutes each night. This is something that has transformed both my own life, and that of hundreds of my students.

Chapter Recap: The Story Inside Your Head

☐ **The narrative is the primary reason we fail.** Overwhelmingly, when we struggle to achieve the same goal over and over, there's an inner story we keep telling ourselves – about why it won't work, why it's impractical, why we just deserve something, etc. Addressing that inner story like "Getting healthy takes a lot of time" is the first step to taking action.

☐ **Steps to overcoming the narrative.**

- Step 1: Pay attention to the narrative
- Step 2: Realize that the narrative is a voice other than your own (so who is it?)
- Step 3: Ask yourself, "Why is it saying that?"
- Step 4: Replace the narrative with new visualizations and affirmations about what you want instead.

☐ **Pay attention to the narrative and change the narrative.** The most important thing here is to understand that there is a voice in our head, *other than our own,* that's telling a story that causes stress, anxiety, guilt, and repetitive patterns of behavior preventing us from succeeding.

Master The Day:
The Million Dollar Daily Ritual

"This is the highest wisdom that I own; freedom and life are earned by those alone who conquer them each day anew."

- JOHANN WOLFGANG VON GOETHE

There's a practice in Buddhism that goes a little something like this: Each day when you wake up, you imagine a little bird on your shoulder that says, "Is today the day? Is it the last day I'll be on earth?" It's supposed to be a mental exercise in living like we're dying: being deliberate about our thoughts and actions throughout the day. Are we saying all the things we need to say to people? Are we being who we need to be, who we *want* to be? Are we doing all the things we want to do? And are we living the life we want to be living? Would we be okay with the way things have gone, with the way the average day goes? If not, what needs changing? It's like the old saying that if you live each day like your last, one-day you'll be right. This practice always struck me as a pretty genius way of training us to be deliberate about how we're living.

But it's bigger than that - and there's an incredible principle here we all can use. When you think about it, life is just a series of thousands of "todays" repeated over and over. Tomorrow is just today, repeated. Wednesday is just Tuesday, repeated. And Thursday is just Wednesday, repeated. Weeks are just comprised of essentially the same day repeated over and over, and then months and years are just composites of the past few months, weeks and days. In other words, if you want to look at where the average person is heading, it's easy: look at what they do today. What we do each day accurately reflects what path we're on, and where we'll be years or even decades from now. It's sometimes a scary, sobering truth.

So if we live today like the epic, finale it's supposed to be, tomorrow will be that way too. And then the week, the month, and the year will all be incredible – better than we've ever experienced. Imagine how good food would taste on your final day on earth? There are very few things to conjure up this feeling, but I've fasted for five days without eating anything, and I'll tell you: I came up with more recipes than Martha Stewart in the dozen or so dreams I had each night. The first meal I ate afterwards had flavors and textures I felt like I had never experienced before in my life. Imagine waking up to the person you love on your last day on earth.

I bet your routine would be a bit different right? You might just lie there for a few minutes, or maybe a few hours. You might just watch them sleep for a bit, whisper things, cuddle them or just stare in wonder. Remember, tomorrow it's all gone. The whole movie is over. *Finito*. The rushed routine of getting out of bed, saying "bye!" without a kiss, and running off to the office would probably change. Imagine it was your last day on earth to see something as ordinary as clouds. You're lying on your back in a park in the middle of a beautiful, perfect summer day. The clouds are light and wispy – you see mythical animals, words, continents and far off places forming in the clouds. You sit down and watch the sunset and watch the sky become electric with pink, purple and yellow hues before the sun sinks below the horizon and the stars come out.

Then you remember: this is the last time you'll ever see this spectacle, so you make sure to take it all in. Can you imagine living a year of your life like this? Or what about a week? What if you just lived an entire day perfectly aligned with the feeling that this really is your last day on earth. Imagine what your life would be like if you did this for an entire year now? Don't you think the entire year would be so off the charts – the smells, the sights, the textures, the love, the gratitude, and the experiences – that it would be hard to replace? What does all this have to do with health?

After applying this this whole idea of the "little birdy," it gave me a kind of daily self-awareness that I didn't have before in life even though I meditated. And it was all because of the emphasis on *this one, small daily ritual that served as a reminder.* So I thought to myself, "Okay clearly this daily ritual anchors in the awareness of really taking the time to smell the roses and enjoy life. But what if I applied to this my health?" It's so easy to begin just about any new habit like meditating, walking, or just eating a home cooked meal a few times a week, but the results don't usually come in the first thirty days. They come in the first one hundred, the first three hundred, or the first 1,000 days. But 99% of us never make it to those first one hundred days.

If we had a magical, crystal ball that could show us a hundred or a thousand days into the future, we wouldn't give up because we would see the progress as time went along. But since we don't have a crystal ball, most of us do give up. For some months I pondered how I could create some kind of daily focal point, a daily routine, much like a monk uses to retain a spiritual or religious focus. Unfortunately, the pieces weren't connecting in my own mind, so I dropped the idea and let it go. And that's when serendipity showed up at the door. A couple months later, I received an email from one of my students who (at that point) was the most successful person that had ever gone through my online program: he was down 37 pounds. Victory!

I was thrilled to hear about his progress, so I emailed him to get some follow up information and find out what principles worked the best for him. At first, we went through the small talk: The nutritional principles, the habits, and the little tiny changes he made to his life to see results. But there was something he mentioned that I couldn't get out of my mind. One thing in particular really jumped out at me, when he said: "I realized that when I just focus on beating *that one day,* the rest of the week seems to take care of itself." I thought about it some more after this conversation – we don't become overweight overnight. We don't eat thanksgiving dinner and magically balloon up thirty pounds, right?

If you asked someone if that's how weight gain worked, they'd laugh at you. You might be laughing now, but we do this all the time. We think that even though we gained thirty pounds over a few decades, we can lose it in two weeks. We think that even though we've had acid reflux for years, if we don't see results *today*, then the remedy we're trying isn't working. We forget that this process had been building, snowballing, and had been underway for months or years. The way out of this is just picking a few small habits, doing them every day, and then being patient. That's where the idea of *"Master The Day"* came from. Because when you think about it, tomorrow is just today, repeated twenty-four hours later. And a week is just today, repeated seven times. So that's why you don't need to think about the weeks, months and years ahead. That's why you don't need to think about spending hours in the gym or loads of time doing things you hate. You just wake up today and make it a damn good day – a few tiny habits at a time. Think about any outcome you want in your life. It's just the result of a few key habits done a thousand times.

Consider the A student in school. What daily habits are they engaging in? Studying each night. Going to study groups. Practicing memory techniques. Organizing their notes. Taking great notes in class. They do that a thousand times, and they're an A student. They don't necessarily study five hours a night (although some do). They just repeat *key habits every day* and focus on being consistent. Think about the happiest person you know. What habits are they engaging in? They take time to always view the positive side of life. They always make sure to express gratitude. They say thank you. They take time to savor life. They do that a dozen times a day, and they're always happy.

Now flip to the opposite side of the spectrum. Consider a really unhappy person. Does an unhappy person possess some magical "illness" that makes them miserable? Usually they don't - they just choose (yes, *choose*, often unconsciously) what daily habits will result in misery and unhappiness. When we're unhappy we tend to choose, 10x a day, blame over personal responsibility. When we're unhappy we tend to choose, 10x a day, to view all the things not working our lives, compared to all the things that *are* working. When we're unhappy we tend to *choose* to wait for 'good timing' to start an important project, rather than starting today. The key part of the "Master the Day" philosophy is that you only need to take your health one day at a time – and all you do is ensure that *today* went perfect.

If you focus on perfecting each day, you have perfect weeks, months, years and decades. And life is filled with skittles, unicorns and rainbows. And weight loss. So how do you master the day? I'm going to give you a five-part daily & weekly ritual. This master the day habit only takes five minutes a day. Five minutes! And here's the best part: it's just a few simple habits you do each day. That's it. Remember that everything we are, who we are, what we are, is just the result of certain tiny habits we do each day, consistently, over time. Swap out the bad habits with the good ones, and as time goes on, life just seems to get better and better. So without further adieu, here's the master the day daily ritual.

The "Master The Day" Daily Ritual

There are five parts to the *Master The Day* daily ritual.

#1 Find your why and write it down.
#2 Visualize the outcome you want.
#3 Visualize the one key action step you're going to engage in today in order to get yourself closer.
#4 Track your key daily habits.
#5 Do the weekly check-in and write out your new habits.

These five steps are the most important part of the book. Don't be fooled by their simplicity. If you read the biographies of many of the most successful people on the planet, you'll notice they do something very similar. Like I said, it might sound weird and unrelated to health ("visualize my why?"), but here's my guarantee, as well as my personal and professional promise: do this every day and in a year you won't even recognize yourself. Your health, and your life, will be incredible. It'll be so off the charts that others won't recognize you, and *you* won't recognize you.

Here's another important side note: you *need to write this down on paper*. Whatever notepad you use, whether it's a physical one or a digital one, go through this chapter, write these things down, and review them each day. So, let's get started.

Find Your Why: Daryl's Story

Daryl was clinically obese since age two. Yes, *two years old*. He was formerly a worker in the video game industry where he spent the days building and testing out new gaming software. There was lots of pizza, lots of junk food and lots of chips. And there was very little emphasis on health or having a thriving social life. There were long hours and short deadlines – all in front of a computer screen. He had many, many physical problems (like taking an *average* of three hours to go to the bathroom each day), but the emotional ones were much worse.

He knew he was never going to get a girlfriend unless he took charge of his health (and his life), because things were looking pretty grim for him. Even his house was a mess – which he told me he later realized was just a metaphor for the state his life was in – total chaos. In any case, one day he realized that his self-esteem had hit an all time low, and he said to himself: *"What the $%&$ am I doing?" Why am I doing this to myself? I feel like crap every day, something has to change now. I can't put this off any longer. I don't deserve this."* At his worst, Daryl was 330 pounds at his maximum weight. These days, he weighs close to 170 pounds. One of the habits I found in *every single one* of those 100+ pound weight loss stories I mentioned was this: they knew their why, and they often had a physical representation of it.

Whether or not they explicitly said, "this is why I'm doing this, and I review it each day" was unimportant – the facts were the same. They all knew what they wanted, and *why they wanted it*, beyond just looking better. Lily, a single mother with two jobs, actually kept an old pair of her jeans from high school when she was a cheerleader. She was committed to fitting back into those. That served as her powerful emotional reminder every single day when she came home. Cindy kept a picture of herself when she was younger. Another woman, Becca, simply had a picture of her mom – who was currently being treated in a nursing home for Alzheimer's – which reminded her of the horrors involved in taking care of someone you love that has dementia. In my own life, clarifying my why has been incredibly powerful too.

Earlier I told you a bit about how visualization helped pull me out of a deep funk in my early twenties. Here's a bit more on the story behind it. After working my first job out of college for a year, I moved to China for a year to study Kung Fu and meditation. The job definitely wasn't my passion, and I figured that if I was going to sit in a cubicle all day for the next forty years, I should probably have some fun now. I had an incredible year in China, but when I returned, at age twenty-four, I had no job, no skills, no friends, no connections, *nothing*. So I did what any sane person would do: I moved back in with my parents (Yeah, about that...). Unfortunately, not long after repatriating to the USA I fell into a deep depression.

The combination of not having a job (and taking six months to find one), not having any close friends, not knowing anyone, and not having a daily routine to keep my mind occupied really messed with my happiness and left me thinking about my purpose and the meaning of my life. One of the most useful exercises that helped me get out of bed in the morning was coming up with a *why*. It doesn't necessarily mean that you have some magical purpose sitting around – if you do, good! But if you're like me and you don't know your why, *create* one like I did - here's how. One other thing: there are lots of different ways to have a "why" that drives you.

Just like I told you about some of these case studies where the people actually had *physical representations* (the old jeans, a picture of their young self, a reminder of something they feared), the more explicit your why is (e.g. on paper) the better. Here's a quick exercise to help you come up with one.

The 20-Minute Brain Splurge

Take out a large, white sheet of people, and get a hold of a great pen. Then make some tea or a nice coffee, and sit in a spot that gets your creative juices going. And then follow the instructions below and *just write*. Don't stop writing until the timer goes off. At the top of the paper write: "Why do I get up in the morning?" and "Why do I want to be healthy/lose weight?"

Just write.

The first 10-20 will be terrible. You'll say stuff like "To live my life fully" and "to live my passion." Those are great, but they won't get you up in the morning when your life has gone to hell. You want visceral, *emotional* things. You want things that stir up fears, or hopes, or powerful dreams that excite you. As you keep doing this, better ones will come out like, "Because being unhealthy sucks" or "When I look at myself in the mirror, I hate what I see." I'll give you some that I've used, and then some that I've heard from my clients and students. I'll start with generic "life-related" whys, and then get to the specific health ones. Often, the two are intertwined.

Here are two of mine:

Write down what you want and why you want it.

What: I want to inspire others by showing them that they can live any life they dream of, if they know want they want and they are willing to work for it. I am going to inspire them through my own story of struggle and then success.

Why: Because I see people around me living miserable lives doing things they hate… and I want to be the exception. Life is too short to live like a lifeless zombie.

Another:

What: My purpose in life is to deliver as much value as is humanly possible to each person I come into contact with each day. Starting with the barista at the coffee shop in the morning, then my coworkers, my girlfriend and my family.

Why: In the end, it's not always easy to control what we *get* in life, but we can control what we *give* – and that can dramatically alter someone else's life.

Here are some health or weight loss related:

What: I want to lose weight and stay healthy because I've seen my mother's rapid descent into dementia and Alzheimer's… I've seen how it can tear families apart, how it can make you crumble inside when your mother doesn't recognize you, and how it can rapidly accumulate medical bills that I can't afford to pay.

Why: I want to take care of myself so my kids never have to worry about this burden, or deal with the emotional (and financial) pain I have gone through.

Here's another one:

What: I want to lose weight because I want to actually like who I see in the mirror again. I'm so tired of getting out of the shower, pausing for a second, and feeling disgusted with what I see and wondering how I got there.

Why: The confidence that losing weight will give me, will allow me to do *all* the things I love again in life – pursue my dreams and hobbies, look great at the beach, and just feel more comfortable in my skin and not have to hide myself from the world, my spouse and my friends.

And one more:

What: I want to lose weight and get healthier because I'm tired of feeling like there are all these things *I can't do* because I feel like crap. I'm tired of being limited by pain and illness, I'm tired of being tired, I'm tired of not sleeping well, and I'm tired of feeling *old*. I'm tired of feeling like all the things I used to love – hiking, golf, gardening, walking the dog, traveling – are off limits because my body is so fragile now.

Why: Losing weight will allow me to do all the things, activities, sports, and travels I love again – it'll help me get my life back.

Finding or creating a why can be incredibly powerful. But there's another reason for coming up with your why – you're going to look at it, read it, and visualize it each morning, and more than just inspiring you It'll remind you of what you committed to, even on the days where you don't want to keep going. For now, circle a few that resonate with you, and keep them on a piece of paper. We'll come back to them soon.

Your Five-Minute Epic Vision of the Future

A few years back, I thought visualizations were a bunch of crap. That's a bit harsh, especially coming from someone who has been meditating since he was twelve years old. I'm open to that kind of stuff. But I've read so many success books and have heard the same old "take action" *blah blah blah* talk, that I didn't really get how visualizations were going to change my life at all, or if they would change my life.

I mean, if something doesn't work, why bother wasting time on it, right? We're all busy. And I thought they were garbage until someone told how me quickly their life changed after they visualized every single outcome they wanted in their life, no matter how far away it was.

So I put it to the test.

For a couple months, I would wake up half an hour earlier, and among the things I would do first thing in the morning would be my visualizations. I took time to look at the different aspects of my life that needed improvement: First, my financial life. I was spending way too much and earning way too little. I saw myself earning more than I needed, saving loads of money, and traveling a few times a year. Then, my health: I was healthy, but recently I was getting sick pretty easily because I was working twelve-hour days and eating fewer plants. Next, my relationship: My girlfriend and I were doing very well, but I wanted to make sure it stayed that way. Then I thought about my happiness: I struggled with happiness quite a lot throughout my mid and early twenties, so I wanted this to be a focus. I spent time seeing myself say "my life is awesome" and feeling like life was good.

Finally, I thought about the bigger picture "dreams" I had: I really wanted to quit my job and change to something new, something I was actually passionate about. I couldn't envision what exactly I wanted here, so I just envisioned myself waking up to a new job or form of work that was enjoyable. I stuck with these five categories for a time, and diligently visualized them every single morning before I left for work. After the first few weeks, there were hardly any miracles. But after a month or two, some interesting things started happening. Friends. A big personal goal of mine was to surround myself with more successful friends. People that were as interested in creating happier, better lives as I was.

So when it came time for my "friends" visualization, I saw myself surrounding myself with friends earning at least six figures in a career or business they loved, with a massive fire to get better in their own lives. I saw us chatting around dinner about our businesses, books, passions, interests, and huge dreams. The first one came into my life within three weeks and we instantly connected. The second one came three weeks later, and the story was similar - we instantly resonated with each other's mission. Where were these people my entire life? I wanted people like this for the last *three decades*, and now in three weeks they magically appeared? Where were they all coming from anyway?

Then I thought about my personal finances. A big problem throughout my twenties, like other youth, was being chronically poor due to my own spending habits. So I visualized myself both spending less, saving more, as well as earning more. But overall, I just saw myself without the stress of worrying about money – which was something that had been a daily reminder in my life for half a decade. Guess what happened? I started magically running into more personal finance people that shared with me their tips and tricks. I randomly (serendipitously) picked up some freelance gigs that brought in a couple extra thousand dollars on the side to supplement my job. A few months later, when I looked back at my bank accounts – I realized I was now saving close to $600 a month – despite earning a tiny income at my day job.

All of this happened without me even thinking about it. The act of visualizing these things changed my behavior in subtle ways that I didn't even realize. At no point did I ever buy a book or take a course on this kind of stuff. It just "happened" because I spent time pondering it each morning.

Then I thought about the state of my happiness. Since happiness was quite possibly my #1 life priority, I made sure that this was the core visualization each day. First, I visualized waking up, and being in a good mood. For some reason, even when everything is going right in my life, I'm always in a bad mood in the morning. I saw myself walking throughout my daily routine with a big smile on my face, and that kind of relaxed feeling you get when you feel like "you're exactly where you want to be, doing what you want to do." I visualized people commenting on how happy and energized I looked, and I visualized the feeling of just loving life.

The strange thing about these visualizations was that I didn't consciously change any of my daily actions. So in other words, I sat down to do these quick visualizations of what I wanted in my life, but I didn't say, "Okay, so today I'm going to talk about three things I'm grateful for, I'm going to meditate, and I'm going to tell the people in my life I love them." It just happened. All of those things in every single aspect of my life that I visualized naturally ended up occurring. You know what the strangest part was? Some time later, after about a year, I re-read the things I had written down on that sheet of paper. And guess what?

Every single one of the visualizations I put down on the paper came true. No I wasn't a millionaire, and no I didn't manifest the winning numbers to the lottery, but it had apparently slightly changed my behavior so much that I was in an entirely different life. Everything that I pondered each morning was now a reality –the new friends I wanted, the better financial life, the great health – everything. "Okay, I get it. You made your point. Looks like there *might* be something here," I told my friend. Secretly, I promised myself that I'd never stop doing this as long as I lived. Unsurprisingly, over the coming months I found out that *Jack Canfield, Jim Rohn, Tony Robbins,* virtually every Olympian on the planet and many – or most - of the world's most successful people regularly use affirmations and visualizations on a daily basis. It doesn't surprise me one bit based on how eerily well it worked for me.

***

Want more proof about how your thoughts and words affect your life? Check out this incredible study done to prove it. **In 1979, an incredible anti-aging study was done.** Have you ever wondered how some people who are sixty seem to be as strong as an ox? As limber as a gymnast? As sharp as a young college student? And then there are some thirty-five year olds that are so sluggish, who appear (and act) twice their age? I became curious, does your thinking have power over your aging, and if so, how much? Can we control it?

A surprising study was done asking this exact same question. In 1979, Dr. Ellen Langer designed a weeklong experiment with a group of 75-year-old men. The men weren't told many details about the study- they were just told they'd be going away on a retreat for about a week at a retreat center. They were not allowed to bring any pictures, newspapers or books dated later than 1959. Once the men arrived at the study, they were told that for the next week they had to pretend that it was 1959 – a time when these men were fifty-five years old. And to make the entire situation more believable, they were encouraged to dress and act like their younger selves, and were even given ID badges with pictures of their fifty-five year-old selves.

They were told to talk about president Eisenhower, and other world events that happened around this time, and magazine issues from 1959 like *Life* were posted around the experiment area. The entire experiment was designed to make them really commit to the idea that they were living back in 1959. Before the retreat, the men were tested in various aspects of their health that got worse with age:

- Physical strength
- Posture
- Perception
- Reaction time
- Short term memory
- Eyesight

Here's what's interesting: **After the study, most of the men had improved in every single category.** They were more flexible, had better posture and had improved hand strength. Their eyesight even improved by an average of 10%, as well as their memory. Over 50% actually *went up in intelligence.* **And this is the best part:** They took pictures before and after the experiment, and they showed the pictures to strangers afterwards.

Guess what they noticed? Random people were asked to observe the age of these men, and the men looked, on average, three years younger than when they arrived. So we know, without a doubt, that our thoughts affect our physical reality. We know that if you think you can become smarter, you will become smarter, and will invest the effort to become smarter. If you think your situation is bad (no matter how it may be objectively) you begin looking for things that reinforce that your situation is bad. How often have you said to yourself, "oh man, I feel old. I'm getting old. I have so many problems. I have so many health issues now. My knees ache, my back hurts, and I need Pepto-Bismol every time I eat."

Just like we know that describing ourselves as happy actually makes us happier, if you describe yourself as healthy, happy and young – you're making real changes. This isn't law of attraction stuff; this is real science in the realm of mind-body medicine. That's how we all know someone who is eighty or even ninety with a very young, child-like spirit, with tons of energy and vitality – they've made a choice to view life as an adventure, rather than a drudgery. There's more to the expression "young at heart" – literally, if we're young at heart, we physically stay younger too. The best part here is that life then follows suit. It's not really a secret that the healthiest, fittest people that maintain good health into old age constantly have this "I'm young at heart" mindset and self-talk. We become what we think about.

***

Okay, back to the visualization stuff. It sounds corny. And I bet it sounds unrelated to being healthy, losing weight, or just being happier. But trust me – there's a reason why the world's happiest, healthiest and richest all do something similar. Here's how visualizing the outcomes you want dramatically changes your life – no belief required. First, it clarifies what you want from life. If you don't know what you want, you won't get it. If you say you want to get "healthier," that doesn't really mean anything, because you can't quantify healthier. Maybe healthier means twenty pounds lighter. Maybe it means feeling light and energetic. Maybe it means sleeping throughout the night. Maybe it means seeing your blood pressure go down.

When you're forced to visualize an outcome, you're forced to think about what you actually want from life, and how you can potentially get it. Think about it, when was the last time you actually sat down and thought, "Okay, what do I want my life to actually look like? What about my body? My health? My sleep? Specifically what do I want each of these areas of my life to look like? What about my relationship? What about my daily routine? My work? My income?" Imagine if you thought about them each day? Don't you think you would slowly begin to make some small changes without realizing it? So the first thing is that visualizations force you to think about what you want. When you think seven days a week about how you want more energy, changes in your behavior happen without you even realizing it. You also begin to think about how you can possibly get there. This is a big shift from living the autopilot lifestyle (AL) where we burn out and complain, but don't spend any time thinking about what needs changing or how we can get the outcome we want.

The second reason this works is a bit more complex. The more we subconsciously think about something, the more we think about how to make it a reality. Way back at my first job as a teacher, I tossed around the idea of starting a business. It wasn't a serious thought, and it wasn't an actual plan, but I was bouncing it around between my ears. "Wouldn't it be cool to have a business and travel whenever I wanted?" Most of the time it was just a re-occurring daydream that occurred on Mondays. But sometimes, I would think about it a few minutes a day. I'd ponder it on my lunch break, and think about it on the way to work. Guess what happened?

Without even formulating a plan, or "wanting" to start a business, I started one. All that thinking slightly influenced my behavior. During my lunch break, I'd borrow a computer in the student library and Google how to start a business for ten or fifteen minutes, rather than check my usual news. When I went to the library in my hometown, one day I decided not to get a fiction book, and instead to get a personal development book. That book led to many more "how to get better" books. And those books and short lunch breaks eventually led to me reconnecting with a friend from abroad, and we started a business together a year later. Even though the business failed, all of this occurred just from a nagging thought and visualization that I didn't drop. And you know, I find this to be the rule, rather than the exception.

When you constantly think and "see" an outcome that you want, something changes in your behavior and your decision making that you can't always explain in terms of logic. It just doesn't exist. It's the same phenomenon that happens when you weigh yourself in the morning. Researchers have actually found that you'll lose weight without changing your conscious behavior, if you weigh yourself daily. In the study, participants were either in a control group, or the test group. The test group was told to weigh themselves daily, and at the end of the week they were sent an email with feedback (and/or reminders to weigh themselves if they forgot to). At the end of the six-month period, the average weight loss in the weighing group was 13.5 pounds. Again, they made no *conscious* changes beyond just weighing themselves quickly.[12]

How?

It's via the same effect. Your subconscious reminds yourself of the new story, "Okay Mike, remember dude, you're trying to cut down a bit. No more doughnuts with breakfast." And even though you aren't *actually* having that conversation with yourself consciously, your brain *is*. So when you go to breakfast or get a quick coffee on the way to work because you're late, something tells you (or helps you) avoid the pastry this time around. You don't know what it is, or how it works, but it does. Something changed your behavior without you realizing it, and suddenly you're losing weight without consciously dieting or doing anything. That magical something is your subconscious – which is powerfully influenced by stuff like this. This is part of that whole "inner game" I talk about.

So, **step two** is to visualize the specific health outcomes you want. Remember:

Be specific. Don't say, "Get healthier." Say, "lose XYZ pounds," or "sleep entirely through the night," or "no longer have knee pain going down stairs."

Here's **step three**: Visualize today's one thing. Now the *third* part of your daily ritual is simple: visualize your one action step for today, and see yourself walking through it. Even though visualizing the outcomes you want in your life dramatically will change your actions in slight, subtle, powerful ways, let's not beat around the bush: you can't wish or pray your way to better health. Sorry, no law of attraction stuff here. It's more complex than that. Only action produces results. No one said it has to be hard (it doesn't have to be), we just have to be consistent. So the final part of your daily (ideally morning) ritual is quite simple. You're just going to visualize one thing you're going to do today. Sure you could list five or ten things, but chances are, the more things you list, the fewer things you'll do. So all you do is visualize one thing for the day, like:

- Walking ten minutes on your lunch break
- Getting up ten minutes earlier tomorrow so you don't have to rush
- Meditating five minutes
- Eating one home-cooked meal
- Avoiding sugar one day of the week

- Changing where you eat lunch one day of the week
- Setting an alarm for 10:50 – the time you should get in bed so you aren't cranky in the morning
- Eating one vegetable today

Boom. No complex to-do lists. No lists of fifteen things you probably won't do anyway. And there's definitely no huge "new year's game plan" to start exercising 4x a week even though we haven't all year.

And now, **step four**: Track key daily habits. Quick side note: I do not mean calories or what you eat, just *daily habits*. So you've got your quick morning routine planned, but now you need reminders. It'd be a lot easier to be successful if you had me sending you a text message every few minutes reminding you to stay focused, but you don't. So here's the next step: every Monday morning, when you sit down at work, you're going to grab a blank sheet of white paper and write down something like this:

```
12/5 Weekly Habits          | M | T | W | T | F |
1. Walk 10 min at lunch

2. Wake up 15 min early

3. High protein with each meal
```

You're going to write out a calendar for the week: Monday through Friday, and then write down whatever habits you're cultivating. It only takes thirty seconds. Ideally stick to just one habit, but don't go over three. And all you do is put a check mark for each day. Make sure to bring this to your work desk since you spend at least forty hours a week there. Wherever you work or spend 40+ hours a week is where this sheet should be. Personally, what I do (since I do this every week) is put a copy right on my work desk (it's my Monday 8:45 am ritual), and take a picture of it so I have it in my phone. And all this does is serve as a reminder throughout the day about the tiny daily habits you are working on.

Remember, it doesn't take massive effort, time, discipline or willpower – it just takes consistency with tiny daily habits. As you go through the week, it's simple: Since this is right at your work desk, you just casually glance at it throughout the day, it serves as your reminder, and then you either do the habit or you don't. And if you do, you put a check mark. If you don't, you don't put anything.

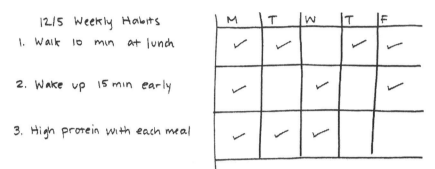

All you're doing is helping you ingrain this idea I call *"master the day."* And to do that, you need constant awareness of what you're working on each day.

Finally, **step five:** The five-minute review. The final step happens each Sunday morning for five minutes. All you do is take out another piece of paper, write down "weekly review" and simply tally up how many times you practiced those habits, like this:

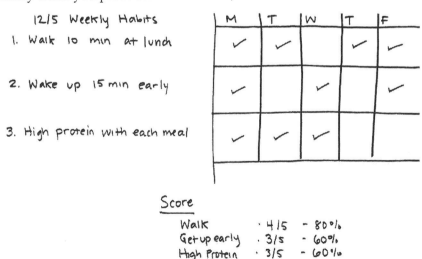

If you did what you said you would, great! Write down what worked. If you didn't, that's fine too – but you need to write down *why not*. You have to get specific, like:

- I didn't make breakfast at home *because* I was too tired and rushed in the morning
- I struggled with sugar because I kept having my afternoon cravings around 2 pm, *because* I was bored at work
- I said I would take my ten minute walk but didn't *because* I waited until after work each day and just was tired and wanted to relax

Finally, write down what *habits* need to happen this week in order to succeed. Write down what new habits you need to cultivate to master the day. Here are some examples:

- *In order to* actually make breakfast a home, I have to set an alarm ten minutes earlier, otherwise I'm too tired and rushed in the morning.
- *In order to* avoid that afternoon sugar binge, I need to make sure to schedule my lunch around that time instead.
- *In order to* actually take my ten-minute walk, I have to either do it before work or do it on my lunch break – because otherwise I'm too tired.

This is extremely important. If something didn't work, we need to understand what habits prevented it from working. Most importantly, next week that new tiny habit becomes the next week's game plan. The weekly review is one of the most important aspects of this. Don't be fooled by the apparent simplicity of it all. Many times when we get frustrated by our lack of progress, or fall into that autopilot thinking, we get stuck because we don't reflect on what is and is not working. "Man, I just messed up that entire week's progress because of John's work party on Friday," we say. But we don't ever reflect on what went wrong. So rather than trying to tackle the *behavioral* reason, we end up just looking for the new fad, diet or plan. But it was never about the plan. Remember, it's about us. It's fine to complain and be frustrated. But it's not fine for us to complain and be frustrated without making changes.

The weekly review (which only takes a few minutes) is so valuable because it provides *insight* into what's not working and why. So if we said our daily habit was to walk ten minutes a day, and we didn't do it a single time this week, we sit down and ask, "okay, why not?" Why didn't it happen? "Well, I always saved it for after work, and after work I'm always tired." Okay, good. That's feedback. That's insight into why it didn't work. So what new habit do we need to cultivate to make sure that it happens this week? Maybe this week I need to do it *in the morning* before work. Or maybe this week I need to do it during the first ten minutes of my lunch break. Or maybe I need a better system for walking *immediately* once I get home.

So, here's the old way: "Man, I never seem to get myself to go for that walk I said I would." And here's the new way: "Okay, It didn't work last week because I waited until after work. Here's a new habit I can try next week: I'll go around the block for ten minutes the first ten minutes of my lunch break, so I know I'll do it while I have energy." Then, this habit gets written down on your weekly review, and put on the sheet for the next week. It makes sense, right? Almost no one does it. All of this only takes five minutes, but the weekly review is critical to understand what's working, and what's not, and most of all: *why* not. So, here's a quick recap of the master the day daily ritual.

The "Master The Day" Daily Ritual Recap

Every Morning:

1. Review your "why" (1 minute)

2. Visualize the outcomes you want – in the present. (1 minute)

3. Visualize the one step you're taking today to get to where you want to be. (1 minute)

4. Track your daily habit(s) with a simple check mark at work and at home.

Once a Week:

5. Do the five-minute weekly review on Sunday, writing down what your *new* habits are to account for where you fell short last week.

Total time every day: 5 minutes.

This is the "master the day" daily ritual. In all of the 100+ pound success stories I studied and interviewed for hours, I noticed different variations on this. The old pair of jeans, having an old picture of themselves, some kind of daily accountability like a friend, journaling about their progress or plans, or some other strategy. The bottom line is that nothing is more effective than daily accountability – a daily ritual. And not only has this process produced wonders in my own life, it has dramatically helped my students and clients too.

This is an easily adapted five-minute morning or evening ritual you can apply (strongly recommend the morning because it's impossible to do in the evening with kids or being tired). Here's the best part: The workload for the entire week to do this? Not even ten minutes a day. Do you think if you spent a few minutes at the beginning of each day to remind yourself, inspire yourself, and visualize the future you want, it'd be a heck of a lot more likely to become a reality? Don't you think it might even be *inevitable?*

Chapter Recap: Master the Day – The Million Dollar Daily Ritual

☐ **The master the day ritual is the most important chapter of this book.** By far, the best way to stay focused throughout the day-to-day, consistent, and motivated is through a *daily ritual*. Typically I have people do this in the morning because in the morning you haven't made any choices yet, so you can "prime" yourself to make the right ones.

☐ **The five steps to master the day** (ideally do this each morning)

1. Step 1: Write down and review your "why" (1 minute)
2. Step 2: Visualize the health, body and life you want (5 minutes)
3. Step 3: Visualize the one step you're taking today to get a bit closer to that vision (1 minute)
4. Step 4: Do the "daily habit tracking" routine every day (1 minute)
5. Step 5: Do the 5 minute weekly habit review on Sunday (5 minutes)
6. Total time: 13 minutes a week, or around 5 minutes a day.

HABIT #3

Wedding Day Syndrome

I find it a bit bizarre. Especially in the western countries like the United States, we're obsessed with weddings. Not marriage. I mean *weddings*. We're obsessed with the dresses, the flowers, the bridesmaids, the bachelor parties, the celebration, the champagne, going bigger and better and making it as memorable as possible. And ironically, despite all this focus on investing tens of thousands of dollars into the wedding day itself, our marriages are dissolving at around 50%. What gives? And what does this have to do with health and weight loss? You'll see in just a second.

One explanation is what I call *Wedding Day Syndrome*, which is one of the fundamental mindset shifts that those 100+ pound weight loss case studies embodied. Although they never described it, this mindset was an unspoken assumption: something they embodied every single day as they strove towards their goal of personal transformation. Wedding Day Syndrome, as I call it, is this: We assume weight loss is an *event*, rather than a *process*. Let me explain.

All over the world, people spend *years* or *decades* preparing for the wedding day itself, which is overly romanticized in movies and in books – and not the *marriage*, which lasts (ideally) decades. In other words, all the hard work is the marriage (one day) – not the wedding. But we emphasize the wedding. We emphasize that one single day when we think it all changes. The same is true of weight loss – many of us have event-based thinking. We think about 'that day' where we look great in the mirror, we go to the beach and people admire us, or the week where we finally lose those thirty pounds for good and look damn good taking our clothes off somewhere. We think about "that day" when we magically have loads of energy, no knee pain, and no more brain fog.

Here's the problem: With event-based thinking, what happens when we get there? We lose our inspiration, and likely quit. So we go on a crash diet for beach season, but then what? We go right back to eating cheesy fries, bacon lollipops and buckets of ice cream. Because we accomplished our mission! "Look great for May 31st on the beach." The other problem is that people with *event-based* thinking tend to create unrealistic lifestyle changes. One time a woman said to me, *"Okay Alex, I'm serious! I'm never eating sugar again. Never. I'm done!"* This is event-based thinking at its finest. Was she realistically – for the next forty years – never going to eat sugar again? No! Not a chance. Could she do it for a week or a month? Probably, yes.

But once we understand that health and weight loss *never end*, we make changes and lifestyle alterations that reflect that. Let me repeat a sobering but secret sauce fact: health and weight loss never end. They just keep going. And going. And going. Until we die. So it's time to start thinking about the process – making realistic changes, making it as enjoyable as possible, and avoiding event-based thinking as much as possible. Once we fully get that health is a process – not a one-time event we magically arrive it – we're already ahead of 99% of people.

Wedding Day Syndrome in Action

Unfortunately, in our "get rich, happy, and skinny in a click" culture, we tend to sometimes forget that happiness, like sadness, usually doesn't just happen overnight. A bird poops on your head? Sure you can be unhappy right now. You inherit a million bucks? Okay, you can be happy for a day or a year. But I mean *the repetitive* state of being unhappy or happy. It rarely happens overnight. It's usually the result of many things, people, events, and mindsets built up over time. So one day we "wake up" and think, "damn, how did I get here? This isn't what I wanted to be doing at this age." We feverishly pursue as many desires as possible. We have our midlife crisis where we move to

Italy, buy a nice car, have an affair, go skydiving, pick up a new hobby, or quit our jobs.

And those things are fine to do. But they never make us happy – and that's because happiness, just like health and weight loss, is a process. Not an event. There's usually no singular event that can make you happy long term, it just doesn't happen. Just like there's no one special thing that'll help you lose thirty-five pounds by next week and keep it off forever. That one's a process. But we kick and scream and get so frustrated. "I want to be happy, *now!*" It doesn't matter how many material things we get once we're at this point. Or even the hobbies we pick up. The places we go. The people we see. None of it matters, *unless we change the process.*

Think back to the core approach. *The Key = The Narrative* + Tiny Daily Habits. Whenever something isn't working, stop looking for isolated events and incidences that caused it. It's almost *never* the case. Instead, look for the process, the habits, and the internal narrative, that created that life over the previous years and decades. Sometimes the habits of the process look like this:

- **Process:** Since I always rush in the morning, I usually get food on the road.
- **Process:** The past few years I've been so focused on my career that I've been going out to business lunches and just eating what's there.
- **Process**: I always took jobs where I valued pay over passion.
- **Process**: I never celebrated my wins, and always focused on my shortcomings.
- **Process**: I always emphasized what wasn't working, versus what was going great.
- **Process**: I've been rushing through life, never taking time to say please and thank you, smell the roses, and tell my partner he/she is seriously awesome.

Remember: The process created it. The Narrative process created it. The daily habits process created it. Events don't cause long-term unhappiness, just like events usually don't cause long-term weight issues over night. We created this over time, and it takes time to fix. What about relationships? Here's another scenario.

Let's say you're middle aged, you're married and you have kids. Your youngest kid is just leaving home to go off to college, and empty nest syndrome is really kicking in. Now that you have all this time alone with your spouse (Gee, when was that last? A few decades ago?) you feel a bit… distant. You don't quite feel as connected anymore. Something feels weird, off, different. Have you fallen out of love? Has the relationship died? Is it time to jump ship? How did this happen, anyway? It must've been because the kids left home, right? They were the glue holding the family together. Is that true? Or was it just the fact that this lack of love was a process building up for years, possibly decades.

In the lover phase, we constantly spend time wooing the partner. We buy each other gifts, flowers, massages, movie tickets and more. And then time comes creeping along, and gradually we get comfortable, content and then complacent. "Well, he sure isn't going anywhere, this is nice!" We tend to do a pretty good job of keeping the spark alive (sometimes), and then kids roll around. And that's when it goes down hill. Between the poopy diapers, the fact that one spouse rarely is as helpful as the other wants, and the fact that one person doesn't want to stay home and miss out on their career, conflict sets in. And a long process has commenced, unbeknownst to the two partners: the primary focus shifts away from each other, to the survival and thriving of the kids. The date nights get less frequent. The flowers and cards all but stop, except for anniversaries. Alone time to express affection is a memory of the distant past. And then we've arrived at today – the last child is gone, the home is empty, and it feels like we're there with a stranger.

How did it ever get this way?

Or was it a process building up so slowly, with thousands of tiny habits, that we didn't notice it until it snowballed? We tend to assume it was the kids leaving or some other magical event. But it wasn't. That was just what ultimately drew attention to the void. Was it the fact that before kids, you got your spouse flowers a dozen times a year – and after kids, only once a year, at best? Just like health, our relationships are processes. The process determines the overall quality of the relationship, and not isolated events.

***

Mitchell is a 48-year-old mailman in his local town in Kentucky. Recently he noticed some health problems cropping up. He started having shortness of breath, poor sleep, mood swings, and some bowel issues. His doc says that he has diabetes and IBS, and that he needs to lose weight pronto. He ignores the doc for a while. Eighteen months later, he starts having some severe stomach and GI pain, and he's passing blood in the bathroom. He goes in for an emergency X-ray and the doctor says, "Bad news, you have a fairly serious bowel disease, and we're going to have to remove part of your colon." Oh, and the *bad* news is that it's going to cost you $25,000. Based on the medical bills, can you tell this story takes place in America? He can't quite figure out what he did that created this condition. He spends an entire week up late at night wracking his brain. "Was it something genetic?" "Was it from last year, from all that fried food I've been eating from the stress?" "Was it because of that time I got sick traveling in rural India?" He can't figure out what thing led up to this. That's because one thing *didn't* do this. A thousand did. A thousand choices this guy made over the course of a few decades, ignoring warning signs like his diabetes, his bowel habits that changed, the more regularly occurring acid reflux, and the sleep issues.

As you can see, it's everywhere in our lives. It's natural and it's human. But now that you've been equipped with this knowledge, you can spot it and purge it before it begins to show up regularly in your life. Remember that everything we want in life, but especially better health and weight loss, *is a process* and not an isolated event. It's a law of nature that a process that developed over time requires another process over time to reverse it. Focus on mastering the process and simply making progress. Whatever it is you want to become exceptional at in your life, become a *process* focused person. Health is no exception: watch out for wedding day syndrome, focus on the process, and the event will be there soon enough.

Chapter Recap: Wedding Day Syndrome

☐ **Health and weight loss are a process, not a magical event we arrive at one day.** Once we understand that being healthy is a process that never ends, we get that any change we want takes time. Becoming hyper-focused on the event only leads to failure and causes us to make unrealistic lifestyle changes.

☐ **Think of health like a marriage.** Approach it *as if* we're trying to do all the little things to build a successful marriage – a little bit each day, being consistent in behavior, etc. We don't just magically one day wake up to a bad marriage, and we rarely wake up to a perfect one – some little daily behaviors led us there. Which ones were they?

☐ **Choices got us here**. Although it may *feel* like one day we woke up in "this bad dream," where we don't even know how we got to the life we're in, if we had a camera where we could rewind and watch every day of our life, the proof was all there – we made certain choices that led us down a certain path. The way back out of the hole is the same way – through being conscious of our daily choices.

Do Less: The 1-Minute of Meditation Challenge

Health and weight loss are almost purely psychological. Remember, that's key #1. The more we begin to understand that it's the thoughts in our head (aka our mental habits) that are holding us back, we understand the game. When you know the rules, it's easy to find ways around them. A few years back, after I came back from living in China for a year, my close friend and I came to a similar conclusion: We loved meditation, including the benefits it gave us in daily life, but it was pretty hard to actually just *sit down* on the damn cushion and do it every day. This enlightenment was hard man. I thought it would be easy.

So when I flew back to the United States and he remained in China, we decided on a challenge – we called It the *One Minute of Meditation challenge*. We both realized that trying to sit down for thirty minutes a day felt great when we did it, but if it was a Friday night, thirty minutes felt like an eternity when all we wanted was to get some pizza and beer. So we made it smaller – so small that we didn't even think it was worthwhile. One minute per day. And then we added *just one minute* each day. That's it. Keep in mind we had been meditating for years already, so thirty minutes was fairly easy. Ultimately, what we wanted was the routine of meditating *at least* an hour a day, every day, to see what kind of health (or spiritual) benefits would accrue.

So even though, if you counted the total time meditating in the first week, we were way under, look at the total time after: Week one with small daily improvements: 1, 2, 3, 4, 5, 6, 7. Total = 28 minutes. Compare that to my old routine, the ambitious goal that was up and down: 30, 30, 0, 30, 20, 0, 0. Total: 110 minutes. On day one, I meditated 30 *times* longer than my new routine! Wouldn't it just make sense just to keep meditating, even If I missed some days? As you can imagine, this is a powerful metaphor for any health or exercise regime you may have. The real results don't come in the first thirty days – they come in the days after those first thirty. Let's look at days 30-90 – where real transformation occurs. This is the real "100 day rule." Take a look at the numbers now.

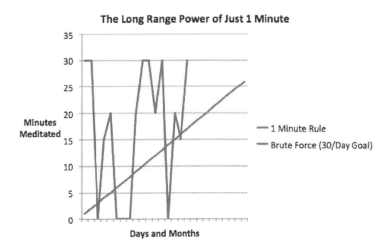

It's pretty clear: on day one, I easily dwarfed the amount of time in meditation compared to if I only did one minute per day. But remember the last chapter's habit: wedding day syndrome. It's a process not an event. And remember the 100-day rule. It's more important to still be doing one minute a day after 100 days, than it is to be doing thirty or sixty minutes a day if it only lasts thirty days. You can see the ups and downs in my brute force "Must do thirty minutes" approach. Some weekends I don't want to. On vacation I might not want to. When I'm tired I might not want to. And that's because thirty minutes seems like an insurmountably large amount of time.

A minute? Just six minutes after six days? I can do that. That's just meditating during a commercial, or while my hot water is boiling to make tea or coffee. Obviously, there's a powerful comparison here. You could easily have swapped out meditation with other daily habits that'll get you closer to where you want to be: Exercise, eating one home-cooked meal per night, eating out one less meal a week, etc. Think about how we often approach our new year's goals. Every single year I'm frustrated (in a selfish way!) because the first three months of the New Year leaves the gym so clogged that I have to park on the street until springtime. Why? The influx of all the people who come fired up ready to change their lives. But I know anecdotally that most of the parking lot is cleared out by early spring – April typically – and research supports the idea that most of us (between 88 and 92%) fail.[13] Here's the thing: It goes against our own psychology.

Inevitably once we've gotten to the point where we desperately want change, we're fed up. The emotional, "ugh, I'm tired of this" has reached a breaking point, and now we want to do something different. In other words, motivation is at an all-time high, and when we're fired up, we can do more than usual. So we follow the typical "New Year's" inspiration and go from zero to a hundred in a week. It will go against every fiber in your mind and body to try and only walk for one minute, or five, or ten minutes. Seriously – you will try to rationalize it and convince yourself that it's worthless and won't benefit you. Ignore the voice – remember that *The Narrative* will begin to get loud. Tell Nancy to shut up, and remind her that you're busy making your dreams a reality.

How Doing Less Will Get You *Better* Results

An interesting study was done with researchers at Columbia and Stanford University that helps illustrate the idea that doing less will actually get you *more*. Researchers wanted to do an experiment (now a famous experiment) on how choices affect our motivation or our ability to take action. The researchers went to an upscale grocery store and put several jams on display at a tasting booth. One booth had either six jams, or twenty-four selections that they could test and check out. The researchers wanted to see how it might affect how many jams people tried, and ultimately, how many they would buy.

Here's what they found: In the booth with the most varieties of jam, more people stopped at the booth (60%), versus 40% who stopped by the booth with a limited number of jams. However, the stand with the most jams only had 3% of the people buy, while the stand with limited jams had 30% buy. That's a 10x difference![14] What's going on here? How's that possible? I'm sure there are many things going on here, but the researchers observed a few things in particular:

1. More jams lead to more shiny object syndrome. The more variety, the more we want to browse and look around without necessarily doing anything.
2. More jams lead to *less action taking*. Only 1/10th of the people actually bought when they had more options, possibly because the options impaired their ability to decide what to buy.

More options = more browsing and less action taking. All of us know this to be all too true. Look what happens when you Google how to lose weight:

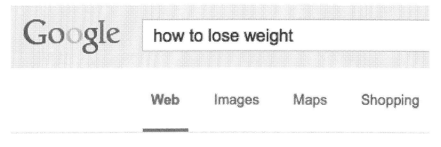

356 *million* search results. It's not really surprising why it's so confusing for most of us. One of the things with this slow and steady, daily approach is that we have to *consciously do less*. Again, it will go against every fiber in your body and mind, but all I'm asking is that you trust the process. It's worked for hundreds of my own students – and probably millions of people all over the world that use these principles without realizing it.

***

So there are two key principles here for this habit. First, choose less. This is the entire idea of just picking a few lifestyle changes and daily habits, and focus entirely on those to the exclusion of everything else. If you're following a specific health or diet regime, just do that! Promise yourself you'll ignore all the shiny objects, dedicate yourself for an entire year to one single approach, and then apply the principles here. If you want ideas, see the "one page food guide" at the end.

Here are a few habits that – done just by themselves – will result in dramatically better health, weight loss, and more. Remember, the key here is *simplicity*. Don't tell yourself that you're going to follow three different health books, one guru, and two personal trainers' advice. Pick a few principles, commit to them, and do them day in and day out. Personally, at a high level, the only real two habits I engage in on a weekly basis are: I go to the gym and lift weights four times a week, for 45 minutes each. I cook 95% of the food that goes into my body, especially Monday through Friday. That's it. And those two things have allowed me to have a six pack for close to a decade now – year round, even when I'm working 12-14 hours a day for years at a time.

There are almost always just a few habits and behaviors that are worth more than all the others combined. Here are a few:

- Pick one day a week, and cook all your own meals
- Eat 30g protein with every meal
- Fill half your plate with plants at each meal
- One day a week, eat for energy (eat vegetarian, no coffee, no alcohol, no sugar)
- Swap out any liquid calories (soda, fruit juice, frappucinos) with lemon water
- Swap out any high G.I. carbs (white rice, white bread, bagels, pasta), for low G.I. carbs (brown rice, wheat bread, etc.)

Each one of these tiny habits (remember – they aren't any special secrets I discovered while doing hallucinogens in South America) has produced *dramatic* weight loss and better health in my clients, as well as people I've spoken with and interviewed. It's just a matter of doing them. And naturally, as you begin doing them regularly, you'll begin doing them more often.

Next, do less. This is the idea behind the one-minute of meditation challenge. In the short run, people with the "brute force" approach may exercise thirty minutes a day or an hour, but they always lose in the 100-day test. The ultimate test is whether or not you can do something for 100 days. That's where the real results start rolling in. On the days when you can't seem to get yourself to do that 30 minute workout, or that meditation or yoga session, or that stretching regime you said you would do, just play this game. Today, only do one minute. The irony is that after doing just one minute of it, it's usually pretty easy to do five, ten, or thirty minutes. The biggest resistance point is beginning. Just like with our meditation challenge, the toughest part is sitting down on the damn cushion to be enlightened!

So, what's your one-minute of meditation challenge? Start today. It's just a minute, right? Anyone could do that.

Chapter Recap: The One-Minute of Meditation Challenge

☐   **Choose less.** We're all overwhelmed, overworked, over stimulated and overstressed. And overwhelmingly, the more things we set out to do, the fewer things we *actually* do. Pick just a few key habits changes – cooking at home five days a week, walking ten minutes a day, quitting soda, and just *commit to those for a year*. Dramatic changes will occur.

☐   **Do less, especially if you aren't motivated.** Fed up with trying to do a sixty-minute workout? Then don't do it. Do just five minutes at home. And if you can't do five minutes, do one minute. It's like this book: if I don't want to write, I tell myself to just write one sentence. The irony is that I end up writing 2,000 words instead. "Starting inertia" is huge – and the way over it is by setting a goal so small it seems pointless, and just doing it.

☐   **The success curve.** Chances are, in the first thirty days, someone who "brute forces" their way through forced workouts every day will see better progress since they're clocking three, four or five hours in the gym. But the real secret isn't the first thirty days, but the first 100. Most of those people quit in the first 100. We're better off doing one minute a day, and working up from there, rather than committing to some huge goal from day one – especially if it just results in guilt, frustration, and *The Narrative* getting all feisty.

I Hate Cardio (& Other Shenanigans): The Power of Positive Snowballs

"Success is not the key to happiness. Happiness is the key to success."

- ALBERT SCHWEITZER

Why bother doing things you hate in order to be healthy and happy? This always puzzled me. There's the "old school" method of health and wellness, which is the "grind it out" philosophy. According to this philosophy, everyone should be given the exact same formula for their health and weight loss, and then if they fail, it's because they weren't disciplined or focused enough. But I always thought this was a bit hilarious. I mean, most of the things I had been successful at in my life, I was successful because *I enjoyed them*, and thus doing them *gave me energy,* rather than *took it away.*

I tried thinking back in my life to a time where I was successful because of pure grit, something without any real purpose or internal driver. I couldn't find one. I decided to sit down in my local inspiration spot and tried to figure out, in the rare situations where I was really exceptional in life, what I did to get there. I went to my favorite coffee shop, got an espresso, and wrote: *things I have been doing for at least a decade.*

- Reading about a book a week
- Lifting weights
- Meditating (on and off)

And then I sat back and thought really hard. Did I force myself to do any of these things? That one was a loud and clear no. It was pretty obvious: we do more stuff we enjoy, and I loved reading, I loved the feeling of energy after lifting weights, and I loved the calm that meditation gave me. That's why I kept doing them. I had done *hundreds* of other hobbies and activities, but they all fell by the wayside because they had other reasons that just didn't drive me. Sometimes I wanted to be good at a skill because I thought it was cool, and sometimes I did things because I wanted to be "successful" and look successful. And sometimes I wanted to do something just because I was bored.

Inevitably, none of those reasons kept my fire burning. So why are these health gurus telling us to just suck it up and force ourselves to plow through the same old grind to get healthy? It didn't make any sense to me. Around this time I came across the field of positive psychology – essentially, how your thoughts affect your actions. I thought about one thing in particular: how to create healthy habits that stick. Creating healthy habits (especially eating habits) that stick is often the toughest part about getting healthy. Anyone can begin, and many of us do begin, but very few people "finish" and stick it out until we get there. But there's a major reason why most people fail. And it's because we take the same old "baby steps" advice, without any real concrete strategies for making that happen, and we ignore the biggest barrier to success: our own psychology.

And this all begins with a highly unethical, bizarre psychology experiment done almost a hundred years ago.

***

Sometimes the biggest barrier to us sticking to the healthy habits we know are going to change our life is simple: we *hate doing them.*

Think about it. For those of us that hate running or hate the treadmill, running on a treadmill makes us want to die. And the thought of it makes us want to throw up, right? Over time we tend to form this unconscious inner association of treadmill = hell. Running = slow, painful death. Running plus the treadmill equals a ridiculously painful death, repeated every day. I fall into this category. I'll pass on any and all running-related activities, thank you very much.

That's not even the problem. The problem is this: as we engage in this emotional, mental behavior day after day, the association grows even stronger. Treadmill. Death. Running. Pain. Treadmill Running. Death. Pain. I hate it. Please no. Stop. Don't want to do this for ten years. And over time, the *association with these kinds of things* becomes almost unconscious and automatic – you can't even get yourself to step in the same room as anyone in the gym, and you can't get yourself to strap on the shoes to go running. So why would you bother doing it? I mean it makes sense; we don't like doing things resulting in pain (e.g. getting injured or burning our hands), and want to do more of the stuff that feels good (sex, eating, sleeping etc.). But for the person trying to get healthy, this represents a unique problem – how on earth can you get healthier, if you hate the very behaviors you have to do each day to *get* healthier?

In the 1920s, an interesting study was done. In the study, the researcher wanted to actually "create" a phobia in a child. Yep, scientists were pretty messed up back then. In any case, he took the boy, "Little Albert" who was about nine months old, and first gave him a bunch of different emotional tests to ensure that he didn't have any pre-existing issues already. He was exposed to a white rabbit, a rat, a dog, a monkey, burning objects and other items. During this examination he didn't show any abnormal reactions – he didn't react to any of them in a fearful manner. He was neutral to them.

Next, he was placed on a table with a white lab rat, and he was allowed to play with it. Again, the child wasn't afraid, and had no problem playing with his new buddy. In the experiment, the researcher showed the rat to Little Albert, and then struck a steel pipe with a hammer behind the child's head, creating a loud nose and causing him to cry. He did this numerous times and an interesting association appeared. After constantly presenting the rat to the child, and then striking the steel pipe causing the child to cry, *anytime little Albert saw the rat (without the sound) he began to instantly cry and move away from the animal.*

So he was actually *conditioned* mentally and emotionally to associate the rat with the horribly loud sound that hurt his ears, even when the researcher didn't make any noise whatsoever. The association became this: Rat = loud noise, pain, and crying. What's even more strange is that he then generalized this response over to other animals and objects as well: when he was shown a dog, a seal-skin coat, and even when the researcher wore a Santa Claus mask with a white beard – he would once again begin crying and try to crawl away from the "sound."

Weeks later, when presented with the rat, this strong phobia was still causing an emotional reaction. This study was a big step forward in understanding how we *condition ourselves* to respond to, or react to things in a certain way. So how can you actually apply this study to your own life, in order to create habits that stick? Those of us that struggle to stick with habits often create *negative conditioning* associated with virtually all the habits we need to engage in to get healthy (walking, eating different foods, going to bed earlier).

Here's how to create a powerful positive conditioning so that you actually look forward to engaging in these habits so you can attain all your goals. Let's take a look at how this stuff works with some examples: Stimulus ==> Response ==> Time (Repeated Application) ==> Mental/Emotional Conditioning. For example, do you hate treadmills? Here's what the association looks like. Treadmill ==> "I hate this" ==> (Done repeatedly, for months) ==> "I don't want to ever do this, so I won't. The idea of treadmills makes me want to die." Finally, the resulting association: Treadmills = misery. Exercise = misery. The gym = misery. Getting healthier = misery.

Here's another example – eating healthy, bland food. What about eating healthy food? I constantly hear from people that they hate the monotony of eating boring, tasteless, flavorless health food meals. First of all, healthy food doesn't have to be bland and flavorless – but we'll cover this in another book. But let's take a look at how the conditioning pattern forms. Healthy Food ==> "This is so boring and tasteless." ==> (Done repeatedly, for months) ==> "I hate healthy food because it's so tasteless, and I don't even want to try anymore." And the resulting association: Getting healthy is agonizing because I have to eat crappy, tasteless food.

One other example – going for a walk. What about just a generic form of exercise and getting the blood going? Let's see how a person can create a repetitive negative mental pattern that stops them from engaging in the tiny daily habits. Walking ==> "This 60 minute walk takes so long." ==> (Done repeatedly, for months) ==> "Walking isn't worth it because it takes so much time out of my day." The resulting association: Getting healthy and losing weight is time intensive, and I can't afford that time right now.

So whenever we get frustrated or fail to stick with the habits we said we'd engage in, we just get that emotional conditioning cropping up saying, "I hate this... this stuff takes so much time, how am I supposed to be able to find time to do this? I have all this other stuff to do..." Obviously, this doesn't help us get to where we want to be. So here's what to do instead. The solution is that we need to build a positive snowball. A positive snowball is a positive psychology term for building positive associations with whatever it is we're trying to do, so that we actually *want* to do it and look forward to it. We see this with anything - our jobs, our spouses, or our health. If you have a job that's constantly stressful, or you have annoying coworkers or a mean boss, after a few months or years you wake up and you are already dreading showing up, right? You've conditioned yourself to hate it. You can feel that pit in your stomach first thing in the morning, even though work is a few hours away.

The same can unfortunately happen in a marriage or relationship. You can begin arguing so much or hating each other enough that *most of your interactions end up negative.*

And then one day, one of the spouses doesn't want to get out of the car and go into the house – because he/she has been conditioned to constantly associate the partner with stress and anxiety. This can go on to be generalized, where seeing the actual house as they drive home starts the anxiety process. Whereas you might have had a positive (wahoo!) or neutral (okay, let's go in) attitude, now you actively dread it. So how do you change it? The whole point is this: changing the conditioning in our mind is critical to being successful at staying healthy. This is what I mean when I say that health and habits are primarily a psychological battle (hello, *narrative!*) Bottom line: we want to look forward to the habits that make us successful, right? If we do, we'll do them more.

So here's how to maintain that positive association. First – stop engaging in behaviors that constantly leave you feeling negative and unhappy after. If a sixty minute walk conditions you to hate walking, take ten-minute walks, or do something else. If you hate going to the gym, stop going to the gym as long, or find another activity you like (Zumba? basketball? gardening? volunteering for an environmental clean up crew?). So the first thing is to pick *health habits* that are at least somewhat enjoyable. This might seem like a strange strategy, and you might be thinking, "Okay, Alex, what if I don't like *anything*?" We'll take about this shortly. But the bottom line here is a life lesson as much as it is a health lesson. Things we actively enjoy doing give us energy, and we tend to do more of them. Things we don't enjoy doing require energy, and we tend to avoid doing them.

This is the foundation behind that whole "find your passion" thing. When you enjoy work, it's easy to show up every day. You actually *want* to show up each day. At the very least, find those things that make you think, "Hmm, this isn't too bad!" Limitless motivation is just as much a matter of choosing the *right* things to work on, as it is about showing up each day.

Second - slice and dice. Just go smaller. One of the biggest barriers to many of us sticking with health goals is the feeling that "I'm just going to fail again anyway, so why bother?" If this sounds like you, by far the most important thing is to set easy goals (not ambitious ones) to accumulate little wins that'll keep you inspired and motivated. This sounds paradoxical, right? On one side, I always encourage people to dream big and visualize huge, insane goals that you have no clue how you are going to reach. However, if you're constantly trying out huge goals that you always end up failing at… you're creating more of a negative association.

You're conditioning yourself to *know* that you fail each time you try a goal, so why bother trying? But if you pick an easily achieved goal, you still get that dopamine high of having achieved a goal. So even if you only walk for sixty seconds, from a long term perspective you're better off having that "high" that builds self esteem, rather than setting a big goal that you obviously didn't get close to achieving.

Finally, the third shift. Make a swap. Let's say you're with your spouse, and a certain activity always generates feelings of unhappiness and resentment for you – maybe your husband never cooks or helps around the home, but when you go out to bowl or have drinks with friends, there's some aspect of his behavior that you really love. In this case, to swap the conditioning ("my husband is lazy and boring"), start doing more activities together where he breaks that conditioning. Start doing the activities where he's interesting, lively, and fun. If his chatty, exciting self comes out when you're at dinner parties – go to more of them – and the conditioning will gradually change.

With your health, swap out everything that makes you beat yourself up. No more punishing yourself for caving on the sweets. No more punishing yourself for lack of exercise, walking, or cooking. No more guilt for missing the weight watchers check in, or some kind of group activity. Walk the dog, and tell yourself you did an awesome job exercising after. Use rewards rather than punishments. Drink one less coffee per day, and give yourself a pat on the back. The result? A positive snowball. This is the same principle I have used to exercise 4x a week, for almost ten years now. I've conditioned myself to emotionally understand that I feel insanely good afterwards, no matter how terrible or tired I feel before. I look forward to it – and *never force* myself to go.

I don't have to convince myself, because I know I'm going to feel great. There's no internal dialogue, debate, or narrative cropping up - I just go, and feel awesome after. As a result this is easily a habit I'll maintain for life (unless something changes), because it's something I look forward to. You can do the same thing with virtually any habit or pursuit in life – but you have to condition yourself or get over negative conditioning. These three things, avoiding activities you actively hate, making it easy to achieve smaller goals, and removing anything that causes you to beat yourself up serve one purpose. The point is not the habit itself – it's maintaining an enjoyable state of mind and positive association. The entire reason for this serves the single purpose of maintaining positive conditioning – actually having you enjoy and look forward to the process.

That's it.

Flat out, there are no techniques, tactics, and secret practices learned from Himalayan monks that are more effective than simply doing something you enjoy. So it's just as important to not only cultivate habits you look forward to – but also to make sure to control *the narrative* so that a negative one doesn't begin forming. Otherwise you're associating all the most important habits (for your success and health) with the hammer being struck behind your head. This is building off that slow and steady approach: go smaller, simplify, do less, and do more things you actually enjoy. Otherwise, you just won't do them.

Chapter Recap: Positive Snowballs

☐ **Follow the energy.** Do things you enjoy, avoid the things you hate. Easier in theory, harder in practice. If you hate doing something (e.g. running), but you know it'll make you healthy, *avoid it if you can.* Instead, focus on activities you find tolerable or – at best – actually interesting. The reason is simple: doing things we hate saps our energy (unless you want to brute force your way through them), and doing things we enjoy can give us energy. What daily habits are the easiest for you to do – while also being effective?

☐ **The positive snowball concept.** The reason for setting smaller, daily, regular goals is because of *The Narrative.* The more we can acquire many, small wins, the more we mentally approach the health and weight loss inspired, happy, ready to roll. The more we associate frustration, repetition, bland food, boring runs with getting healthy, the less likely we are to actually *do* those things we said we would.

The Benjamin Franklin Method of Actually Achieving Our Goals: The Power of Rituals

He would start the day with coffee – which he prepared himself after meticulously counting out sixty beans per cup, and by counting them one by one for the perfect dose. In the afternoon he would compose his music, in the evenings he would drink wine and enjoy a leisurely dinner, and afterwards would go for a long, vigorous walk all the while carrying sheets of music paper and something to write with. Afterwards, he'd stop at a tavern to read the news, and then again have another simple meal followed by some beer and a pipe. Then he'd sleep and repeat it all over again.

Doesn't sound too special? This is one of the daily rituals of one of the most brilliant composers in human history: Beethoven. Mason Currey talks a lot about how many of the biggest names in the history of creativity have similar daily routines, in his book *Daily Rituals: How Artists Work*. For example, he talks about how Victor Hugo would wake daily from a gunshot by the nearby fort, have coffee, and have two raw eggs before having his public ice bath on the roof. Balzac, the famous French writer would write in manic episodes, fueled by as many as 50(!) cups of black coffee each day. Sigmund Freud would see patients in the morning while smoking as many as twenty cigars each day, and then go for a power walk around Vienna in the afternoon (something that a surprisingly large amount of creatives do).

Charles dickens would write in his personal study (in perfect quiet) before taking his long, brisk walk through London or the surrounding countryside. And Benjamin Franklin would take time each day in the morning to figure out his own resolution for the day, plan the coming day, work, and then in the evenings reflect on his daily virtues and values: "what good have I done today?" It wasn't until I began searching for how the "best" master each day, that I finally stumbled upon one of the biggest success principles on the planet. Monday can roll around and we're fired up and excited to begin. We start making a home made breakfast, we take that time to walk for ten minutes, we go to bed a few minutes early, and we celebrate our victory. That was easy!

The week progresses and the most deadly day of the week arrives – Friday. It's a friend's birthday, and everyone wants to go out to get drinks, and there's loads of pizza and beer. You're doing a great job dodging the minefield of junk food but Peer Pressure Pamela chimes in and says, "oh, live a little" and guilt trips you into eating. It's all down hill from there. You binge on everything around and break your regime for the first time all week. You wake up the next morning, and feeling like you just destroyed your past week's progress, wonder if it's even worth trying again – is it even worth starting over? Noticing how common this cycle was in my own life and that of my clients, I really spent time wondering about how to address it.

How could I dodge the minefield of Friday nights, friend's birthday parties, social events, and business lunches? What special something, besides my habits or using sheer discipline, would actually allow me to do the stuff each day that I *said* I would? And that's when I stumbled upon a principle that virtually all of the world's most successful utilize on a daily basis: rituals. I already introduced you do the "million dollar *Master the Day* daily ritual," which is a super easy way to hold yourself accountable, stay focused, inspired and motivated every single day. But what happens when you're in the thick of things? What happens when it's a Monday afternoon and you're exhausted, and you *know* you shouldn't eat that sugar snack but you also *know* it's going to make you feel a heck of a lot better? It all starts with a book, or rather, an author.

"There are certain things I do if I sit down to write," he said. "I have a glass of water or a cup of tea. There's a certain time I sit down, from 8:00 to 8:30, somewhere within that half hour every morning," he explained. "I have my vitamin pill and my music, sit in the same seat, and the papers are all arranged in the same places. The cumulative purpose of doing these things the same way every day seems to be a way of saying to the mind, you're going to be dreaming soon."

- STEPHEN KING,
QUOTED IN *HAUNTED HEART:
THE LIFE AND TIMES OF STEPHEN KING*[15]

This can seem a bit strange to some of us. I used to view creatives as these muse-inspired, fly by the seat of their pants, write only when inspiration strikes type folks. But the more I investigated the best of them (not just authors), the more I realized the exact same truth: rituals, routines, habits and little disciplines ran their success – not just random, muse-inspired sketches and drawings. The idea of the accidental creative, just writing when inspiration struck, was blown out of the water. And that's when I realized that virtually anyone at the top got this simple truth too: that rituals and routines are the cornerstones of consistency.

Check out this snippet of the interview I mentioned way back on the chapter on discipline. Here's what Michael Phelps' trainer said about his regimen:

"All he needed to do was target a few specific habits that had nothing to do with swimming and everything to do with creating the right mindset. He designed a series of behaviours that Phelps could use to become calm and focused before each race, to find those tiny advantages that, in a sport where victory can come in milliseconds, would make all the difference. When Phelps was a teenager, for instance, at the end of each practice, Bowman would tell him to go home and "watch the videotape. Watch it before you go to sleep and when you wake up."

***

So how can we actually set up daily rituals that make us as effective as an Olympian or Stephen King… while still allowing us to have fun, eat what we want, and do what we want? There are a couple ways. When you have some tiny habits you want to practice, here's how you can ingrain them in your daily schedule. You can set up rituals based on time, based on the day, based on location, or based on emotional anchors. So let's talk about these now.

First, set up rituals based on time of the day. Here's the biggest "time-based" ritual that has transformed my life: my morning routine. Since it's changed my life so quickly, and has helped many of my students and clients, that's why I chose it as a major focus for this book. And the reason I can do it consistently so many days of the weeks is because it's ritualized at a certain time. So the habit is linked to a time period of the day. And after awhile, just like not brushing your teeth or taking a shower, you feel "weird" starting your day without it. That's exactly what you want. I know that when I wake up and the alarm goes off, the first thing I do is drag myself out of bed, put on warm clothes, and drop down and set my alarm for ten minutes to do some yoga.

Yoga wakes me up and triggers the next phase of my routine: meditation. Once I've warmed up, and I'm awake, and my heart is pounding, I know I won't fall asleep. I sit on the same cushion in the same place. Once my alarm goes off for meditation, I know it's time to get out "the sheet." "The sheet" has my purpose on it, my why, and it says in the exact order what things I should do based on my *Master the Day* daily ritual. Step 1. Step 2. Step 3. Step 4. Remember – systems are the way to success. So I just go through my system. Review my why. Visualize the better future I want for myself (health, wealth, happiness, relationships, meaning, purpose), and then I spend a few minutes reading an inspirational book guaranteed to put me in a good mood no matter how I feel now.

Finally – I sit down for just 30 seconds and remind myself, "This could be the last day you get. Make it count – and that doesn't just mean work hard. It means focus on what's important." Here's the thing: I now feel weird, like my day is off, without doing this routine now. On the weekends when I just want to get out of my apartment, it feels uncomfortable doing this, like there's something important missing. The habit – this morning system – has been so deeply ingrained because of the time of day that I have linked it to. So timing is just one powerful way to anchor in new habits and behaviors. If you've been struggling to really solidify in a new habit, pick the same exact time to do it every day and make sure you actually do it. Write it in your calendar, set a reminder on your phone, and then make it happen.

Next, set up rituals based on the day of the week. One of the "rude awakenings" I got in my early twenties was about personal finance. I got my first job where I wasn't earning too much, pretty much was buying whatever I wanted, and naively assumed that since I "wasn't buying lots of physical stuff" I probably had loads of money left over. Big mistake. I woke up one day to a bank account that said $-54.76, wondered how it was possible, and then went through my bill and realized that I spent $400 on restaurants and bars that month. Ouch. How was I actually going to stop this from happening though? I definitely *was not* going to be that guy recording every purchase, keeping receipts and making my wallet five inches thick, writing down everything on a notepad.

Side note: remember *The Narrative?* I had a pretty big one behind financial stuff. I didn't want to act stingy in my daily life because I didn't want my friends to think I was poor or didn't have any money. I wanted them to think I was doing okay and didn't really have to worry about petty dinners like $20 tacos and a drink. So the story for me was *fear of criticism* and wanting to fit in and look good. Once I honestly had that conversational "aha" with myself, I could go on to change it. So I picked one tiny habit: Every Sunday morning, I had to spend ten minutes writing down the major spending categories (accounting for 90% of my money spent), on a piece of paper, and then take a picture of the paper to save it. That's it. I would use mint. com to track my overall expenses, auto sort them into categories, then just copy that picture down on a piece of paper.

Sure enough, guess what happened after a month or two of this? Sunday mornings became personal finance mornings. And after that time, it was pretty easy to actually keep up with this ten-minute habit of quickly doing my finances, comparing the numbers, and then not freaking out during the week. Obviously, my expenses dropped dramatically, I started saving money for the first time in my life, and I was a lot less stressed. So how can we use this for our health? Well, later on when I wanted to cultivate very specific health habits, I used Sundays for my fifteen-minute reviews, and just like my finance day, they became a habit. I'd go to my favorite spot – a corner in my favorite café – and instantly it would trigger the routine because every Sunday, around the same time, I would do the same thing.

For my own personal goals, regarding the *master the day* routine, I would just look at my daily habit sheet for the week, see what percentage of the time I reached them, and from there I would write "what worked?" and "what didn't work?" Then I would just write down one sentence about what needed to change next week. So going back to my meditation example, I looked at my daily "master the day" sheet, realized that only 3/7 days I successfully meditated, and then asked myself why I only did it 3/7 days a week. Certain repeated themes came up like:

- "I waited too late in the day, and by that time I realized I wasn't going to do it" (Solution: Do it earlier in the day or in the morning)
- "It was the weekend and I really wanted to get out of my house and do something fun" (Solution: just do it during the week)
- "I was rushing to the office too much and couldn't calm down and set aside the time to really make it happen" (Solution: go to bed 15 minutes earlier, so that I can get up 15 minutes earlier without stressing out)

So over time this weekly ritual of sitting down on Sunday, assessing what worked and what didn't (and why), became a million dollar ritual for me because I finally did it after years of not sticking with the habit. Creating rituals based on the day of the week is one powerful way to sets anchors and triggers that become automatic after a time. You can also set up rituals based on location. For almost a year now, there's a great coffee shop where I live that really gets the creative juices flowing. It's ten minutes down the road from my house, and it has that indie vibe, where it's not quite as corporate, plain and stale as a franchise but there's funny stuff on the wall, large windows with natural sunlight, and a cool overall feeling to it.

For the past year, I've gone right from my job to the gym, to this coffee shop until they close at ten or eleven pm. Usually most weekends I'm doing the same thing (especially as I write this book). The strangest thing happens when I arrive there though: I want to work. It's weird, and I can't quite explain it. But the ambiance of the place makes me want to write and create and not procrastinate. It doesn't take any convincing or forcing myself. I just show up, and think "Wow, I really want to read a book or write a book right now." Naturally, as I get to the coffee shop, I get my espresso, sit down, look out the window for a bit, and then my ritual kicks in: this is my writing spot. Or this is my reading spot. Or this is my "think about life" spot. So think about what kind of location you can potentially set aside for one of your habits.

Maybe one of your tiny habits is going to be reading five pages of a health book per day, to remind you of what you're working on, to get new ideas, and just constantly keep your subconscious focused on the fact that you're working on your health. You could pick a good corner of your house, a local coffee shop, the first five minutes of your lunch break at your desk, or somewhere else on the weekend. Eventually, after a few weeks, *it feels weird* not to do it. Jackpot. That's when it all becomes automatic. Pick a good location that you want to use as a trigger to anchor in a specific habit.

***

Now you know that Bestselling Authors, Olympians, Business Magnates and many others all have rituals that allow them to function optimally throughout the day – and that's because *they work*! So how can you apply this in your own life?

Lily's Story: The High School Jeans Memento

Lily, one of the 100+ pound case studies I talked about near the beginning of the book, was a cheerleader in high school, but as she was going through graduate school as a single mother with a job and a commute, she had virtually no time left for herself at the end of the night. As a result, her ordinarily slim cheerleading weight of 120-130 pounds ballooned up to close to 220 pounds – about a hundred pounds over her natural bodyweight.

Around the time when emotionally it began to take its toll ("I was too embarrassed to even go out with my high school friends because I didn't want them to see what I had become"), she had a smart strategy. She pinned up her old pair of high school jeans on the wall in a clear spot in her bedroom. First thing in the morning, that's what she looked at. Last thing at night, that's what she saw. Sure enough, this powerful daily memento (or reminder) anchored in that desire for her "old" body, and reminded her every single day of her goal. A few years later, she ended up fitting back into those exact jeans, and lost the majority of the 100 added pounds in a year. This is an example of that final category – an emotional anchor. Mix this with a specific location or time (like Lily did), and you've got a permanent source of motivation and inner focus. Most importantly, *each day* it'll reinforce and re-affirm what you're working on and trying to do here.

What can you use as an emotional anchor? Sometimes that's as simple as reviewing your "why" each morning, and sometimes that can be as simple as looking at an old picture of yourself each day, or a picture of someone else you aspire to look like.

The Don't-Punch-My-Boss Lunch Break

One of my clients was a stressed out businessman working in the finance industry with a real jerk of a boss. Because of my client's daily routine (read: ridiculous hours), he had minimal time to do anything for his health if he was going to still keep his job, commute to it, and see his family before the weekend. In other words, with the insane hours, he didn't have lots of wiggle room.

When I offered suggestions and strategies, he almost inevitably shot them down with the default "I have zero time" response. So I brainstormed and finally came up with something simple: he said his boss constantly was stressing him out, he needed exercise (but couldn't find time), and he was constantly eating a stressed lunch at his desk. We settled on one tiny habit that kick started everything for him: he had to actually take his lunch breaks, and spend the first ten minutes walking around the block. That's it. Fresh mind, fresh air, exercise, getting out of the office, not having to deal with his boss, no more indigestion from eating and working simultaneously, and lots more. And you'd be surprised how quickly this spilled over into other aspects of his life.

Yeah he cleared his mind. And yeah he got some fresh air, stress relief, and some exercise. But what he really understood was how much a tiny ten-minute habit could make him feel incredible and really change the course of his day. That day his mindset shifted: he now understood that succeeding at getting healthy or losing weight had little to do with forcing yourself to eat less or move more, it was fundamentally about altering the thousands of tiny choices we make each day, and avoiding the autopilot lifestyle (AL). So for this person, it was also a time based habit. He chose the same time each day where he could "activate" the habit.

The Water Break Ritual

Last year, I noticed myself getting painfully dehydrated around the same time every night before bed. I was going to the gym four days a week, training judo three days a week, and otherwise working lots of hours at my job. In general, I was really over doing it, but in particular, I was physically overdoing it and not taking the rest required for that much training. But the constant thirst and brain fog was bothering me lots. I knew I was dehydrated, because I was sweating like a beast after each judo class, and I made sure not to drink water before so I wouldn't cramp up. Each day I promised myself, "Okay Alex, remember to drink more water today, otherwise after Judo you won't be able to sleep again."

Every day, like a perfectly normal human being, I started off with a glass, but pretty much didn't do anything else. I knew that I had to get off my autopilot lifestyle and create a ritual and habit behind it. So here's what I did: At my office, there was a water filter and water cooler in the room next to mine. I tried bringing in water bottles each day to fill up, and I just kept forgetting to fill them up, leave them on my desk, or I left them in my car or lost them. So instead, I put the actual filter and cooler on my desk. It didn't matter if it was full or empty, even though it was a handheld filter; it was so painfully large on my desk that it was obviously around me all day.

Throughout the day it reminded me to go to the kitchen, fill it up, and then put it back near my desk. And since it was there, I ended up drinking it anyway. After just a week of this, I didn't have any more dehydration or brain fog, and finally fell asleep quickly after training. This is how to anchor a habit to a specific location. Let's say you're trying to also trying to drink more water, or maybe you just want to make better nutritional choices. Anchoring a habit to a location might mean one of the following:

Use the refrigerator. Cover your entire refrigerator with a picture, reminder, or object that focuses you again, so any time you want to go get food out of the fridge, you have the reminder right in your face. Or you can go a bit more extreme: putting the scale next to the dinner table or *in front of* the refrigerator. A friend personally used this, so any time he went to eat food he had to step on the scale first, which naturally influenced the decisions following that.

Anchor in a work ritual. If you're struggling with productivity, create a work ritual around your physical desk. It can begin with thirty seconds of cleaning up, one minute of writing down what you have to accomplish today, a few minutes to get or brew your coffee, and then sitting down around the same time. This is the ritual that Stephen King talked about, and many other creatives use as well. This is why morning health-based routines work so well and why many business executives find themselves exercising first thing in the morning. So now you realize that rituals are one of the best ways to anchor in new habits, with minimal discipline and willpower, and to go on and master the day. Pause and think for a moment about what habits you can set up to be anchored to a specific *time* of the day, a specific *location*, a specific *day* of the week, or even a specific kind of motivational, emotional reminder you can look at every day.

Chapter Recap: The Power of Rituals

☐ **Something every day.** Many of the greats in the world – authors, Olympians, business people – bypass willpower and discipline by having the "do something every day philosophy." The one I suggest here is a bit less hardcore: The something every day doesn't have to be six hours a day of exercise – just make sure you do something. After that, you can go to bed guilt-free, even if you didn't run for the half hour you said you would.

☐ **Anchor in habits based on rituals.** Let's say you have a new habit you want to cultivate: reviewing your progress each week. You could randomly choose a time or place to do it, but the best way to make sure it happens is to ritualize it based on:

- **The day of the week** – for example, weighing yourself every day.
- **The time of the day** – for example, having a morning routine where you get clear on what you're doing today to take one step forward. Or during your lunch break, taking the first ten minutes to go for a quick walk.
- **Location** – for example, I keep the water cooler on my actual desk, and I naturally end up drinking more water.
- **Emotional anchors** – for example hanging your old pair of jeans (or a picture) in a prominent location in your bedroom or office like Lily did.

HABIT #7

100 Days of No Goals

"Don't aim at success. The more you aim at it and make it a target, the more you are going to miss it. For success, like happiness, cannot be pursued; it must ensue, and it only does so as the unintended side effect of one's personal dedication to a cause greater than oneself."

- VIKTOR FRANKL, HOLOCAUST SURVIVOR

Despite the fact that we're mostly talking about weight loss here, I want to tell you my story about my own weight struggle. This might sound strange and a bit unrelated, but I have struggled with trying to gain weight my entire life. "Oh, what a lovely problem to have," you might be thinking. Unfortunately, it's not really the case. There's an important lesson here in why most of us fail to achieve our goals – and why we drive ourselves miserable getting there. For a young *man* in his twenties to have a *female* supermodel figure is about as damaging to a young man's self-esteem as it gets.

No, really, it doesn't get any worse. At around six foot two I was 135 pounds – the heaviest I had ever been, and I was twenty-three years old. I was a fully-grown man, taller than most, weighing in at a whopping 135 pounds soaking wet. Let me be perfectly transparent here: there aren't many women that want to date a man that weighs 135 pounds. It's almost like dating a child – someone they feel like *they* have to protect, not necessarily someone that can protect them. After quite a few decades of being unhappy, single, and underweight, I set a very clear goal: I needed to gain twenty pounds. So I did all the stuff I was supposed to do. I made sure I was lifting weights four or five times a week. I made sure I was eating much more than normal. I made sure to eat burgers and all kinds of things at home, including whatever was in site. But like most of us, I was hardly making progress, and my weight was hardly budging. I saw myself getting a bit fatter around my waist, but my muscles and rail-thin legs weren't gaining the real mass I wanted to look normal.

To be honest, the longer I did this, and the less I saw results, the more I became discouraged, frustrated, and starting getting pissed off at the world. And the more I disliked myself. After getting discouraged a dozen times a day, I realized one thing: It was going to take me a lot longer than I thought it would. I started around my early twenties, and it wasn't until age 25-26 that I ended up getting up to 150 pounds. So the only thing that ended up happening was that I gained a bit of weight, but I ended up looking in the mirror more frustrated than ever because after all that work I was still so damn skinny and resembled a woman more than a man.

I still got those comments that my friends & family didn't mean to be hurtful, but they were: "Hey string bean!" "Wow, you have tiny wrists." Another person said, "you're such a skinny lad, you need to lift some weights," despite the fact that I had been lifting weights as long as the biggest guys in the gym. Over time what happened was overwhelmingly negative. I was grumpy all the time, because I hadn't "hit my goal" even though I made progress and had gained a decent amount of weight (I was around 150 pounds at that point). I had noticeably made a lot of progress, but I just wasn't where I wanted to be. And like most of us, I was only good at looking at what I didn't like, rather than what I did like. I felt like a failure. I was disappointed.

I didn't want to repeat this goal-setting and failure process over and over. And I was discouraged. "I do all this work, but *why even bother?* I'm going to keep hating myself if I look like this forever."

***

It wasn't until some years later that I realized that this is pretty much how goal setting goes for most of us humans on the planet. It goes terribly. We set an ambitious goal because we want to improve our life in some way. Ironically, the only thing that ends up happening is that we hate our daily life because we're constantly comparing it to the goal of "am I there yet, or not?" Progress apparently doesn't matter. Neither do results. Just achieving the goal matters.

What happens with this kind of narrow focus? This thing that originally was there to improve our life, ends up making our quality of life worse. It makes it infinitely worse. We get obsessed with the end point, and forget the day to day. We ignore the day to day (also known as "life"), because only the goal matters – that one event in space and time where we can say, "I made it!" What a joke. Some time later I finally did an experiment. My own perfectionism and striving for achievement was making me sick: physically and mentally. In my mid twenties I had some lovely experiences resembling panic attacks and anxiety (almost constantly) because of my self-imposed pressure to "achieve my goals" and finally realized a profound truth: It's better to enjoy life. And it's better to enjoy life without stress and anxiety so bad you want to jump in front of a bus to make it stop. And you know the fastest way to do that?

The fastest path to happiness (and ironically, achieving your health goals) is to stop setting goals and focusing all your time on them. Now, *hang on just a sec.* You're probably thinking, "Don't set goals?! How am I supposed to *achieve* anything in my life? Didn't you just tell me to set huge goals that inspire me?" We'll talk about this in just a second, but here's what happened when I stop tracking goals (and tracked another metric instead). You be the judge of the results.

First, I had zero stress or anxiety each day. Zero! I went from nut job to Zen monk pretty fast. I was never in a rush anymore. I was never overwhelmed. I never had deadlines, so I never had that time crunch pit in my stomach. I sat back, unclenched, and finally began enjoying life again. Paradoxically, I also achieved more progress towards my goals in the next year, than I had in the past five. For those of you who are constantly overwhelmed, stressed to the point of explosion, who have no idea what "quality of life" even means, you'll really appreciate this. If you wake up and life is Monday, then suddenly Friday, every single week for years and decades, then you'll *really* appreciate this even more.

Here's the best part: I achieved more than I ever did with goals. The problem was that my stress, anxiety, perfectionism, and self-pressure prevented the most important part of goal setting: growth and learning. And ironically, paradoxically, once I removed the reason for stress, I grew, applied, and learned much quicker than ever before. This flies in the face of most of what we know about "goal setting" which is an extremely western, logical idea. Set a S.M.A.R.T. goal and achieve it right?

Wrong.

Look at the New Year for proof with millions of people every single year. Apparently we don't really taste our own medicine, because we keep doing the same thing. Only 8% even get remotely close to their goal. What about the other 92%? We "fail." What's worse? We internalize the failure. "Every single year I fail to achieve my goals" is the story, which then goes on to become a full-blown narrative, the backstory of our life: "I always fail to achieve my goals." That's when it becomes scary, because that's when we stop trying and fall into that pit of helplessness where we don't even bother trying anymore.

Goals create black or white space in our thinking, when in reality almost nothing is black or white. Goals say, "You either achieved this or you did not, and you can't relax until you're there." Partly, that's what makes them effective. You either hustle until you're there, or you don't. And that's great "rah rah" motivational B.S., but for most of us it just isn't realistic. It does more harm than it does good. Drop the goals, and the narrative quiets down. You can start and stop as many times as you want, and keep making incremental progress without losing your sanity or self esteem. I'm going to introduce you to a system shortly for both having goals, but not letting your happiness and very existence hinge on whether or not you're "there" yet.

Succeeding Without Goals

If I have no goals, then what on earth do I focus on? How do I achieve anything or make any progress? I was first attracted to this idea when I was reading Eastern literature, the Taoist and Buddhist ideas, where there's a big emphasis on "non-action." It's the idea (or observation) that in nature, nothing is forced or rushed; yet everything works out, as it should every single year without fail. No stress. No anxiety. No problems. Now that's great and all for nature, but I've got stuff to do! I'm on a timeline here. I figured, "what do I have to lose?"

I decided to just try it out. I would have the goal – and it would be on paper – but I would rarely set deadlines for it. Sometimes the only deadline would be "you have to work on this for one hour a day" but otherwise there were no "get X done in Y time" type deadlines. I needed something that I actually tracked each day, so instead of tracking progress towards the goal (output - the end result), I just tracked input. All I tracked was what I did each day, which *habits* I did each day. So the entire approach literally flipped itself 180 degrees. Here's what that looked like. Old goal setting: lose ten pounds. "This week I realized I'm only 12% towards my goal. I've got a long way to go." New goal setting: lose ten pounds. "Today, and this week, I did 7/7 habits I said I would to get myself there. Victory!"

Are you seeing the difference? The first goal creates stress and anxiety and disappointment. It introduces pressure. It's focused on the gap – where we are versus where we want to be. The second one creates positivity. It emphasizes what's working. It emphasizes the present. And here's the kicker: on both "goal charts" I was equally making the same progress objectively. It was just a matter of how I viewed it. I then applied this to any other aspect of my life. Rather than tracking progress towards the goal, the only thing I tracked was the key daily habits that would get me there, and whether or not I did them every day.

That's how this idea of "master the day" came to be. I learned that if I only mastered each day (did the habits I said I would), not only would I reach my goal faster than ever before, I would do it without stress, anxiety, disappointment, guilt and self-hatred. Here's how you can apply the same - if goal setting has been driving you mad, and to higher levels of unhappiness and guilt.

***

Here's what you need to know. First, despite all this you should set the goal and make it a huge one. Make it big, make it unrealistic, and make it incredible. We talked about this earlier, because the very act of setting a large goal requires you to think differently than you ever have before in life – which is where the biggest self-growth comes from. Setting huge goals also inspires you – much more than saying "I'll lose a few pounds this year." Second, you should have that goal on paper and you should see it and read it each day (See the chapter on *Master the Day*). Then, forget it.

Here's what you do instead to track your progress towards it day by day. Think about which habits are going to get you there (pick just a few). Track the daily habits. And then do the weekly review. That's it. It sounds insane, but trust me, it works *way* better than setting goals, and best of all: it doesn't run you ragged trying to achieve them. So here's what that looks like instead.

Old goal setting: "I want to lose twenty-five pounds, and I've only lost two pounds, I have twenty-three pounds to go, so I'm going to be a ridiculous ball of stress and anxiety until I'm there. I can't relax and unclench until I've arrived."

The problem: My thinking is stuck in the future – not in the present. "Oh man, why have I only lost two pounds this month? This is total crap. It's not working, and it's not working fast enough, I'm never going to get there, I hate this stuff…"

New goal setting: Master the day + whatever daily habits I set for myself that week. So I do the quick focus routine in the morning, and the *only thing on my list today*, the week, the month, and the year, is to check off the daily habits, and at the end of the week tally them up.

Monday: Did I drink four glasses of water, take the probiotic and sleep thirty minutes earlier? Yep! Check.

Tuesday: Did I drink four glasses of water, take the probiotic and sleep thirty minutes earlier? Yep! Check.

Wednesday: Did I drink four glasses of water, take the probiotic and sleep thirty minutes earlier? Nope! Sad face.

Thursday: No.

Friday: Yes.

Saturday: No.

Sunday: No.

So I stuck with the daily habits 3/7 days or around 43%. Now I know – in real time – just where I will be a year from now. If I only did 43% of my daily habits, I'll only be 43% of the way towards my goal at the end of the year. Is this stuff starting to make sense? Rather than each day focusing on the progress bar, you're still focusing on the goal, but rather focusing on the lack ("I'm only 2% of the way there, and have 98% to go"), you focus on the day ("I did 3/3 things I said I would to push myself forward").

There are a number of huge benefits here: First, it keeps you focused on the present. You've probably heard that old meditation quote that goes something along the lines of: If you're stuck in the past, you're depressed. If you're living in the future, you're anxious. Traditional goal setting keeps you locked in the past ("I always fail" – depressed), or the future ("Oh man, I'm not on schedule to reach this goal. This sucks. What's going wrong? Not… fast… enough…" – anxiety). This new method has you focused just on making progress in the present, rather than where you are on the timeline.

Remember, the more you think about the outcome, the more you ruin the present because you get sucked into the drama of past and future. That reinforces *The Narrative*, which only makes it that much harder to be happy, content, and successful reaching your goal. The fastest path to getting to where you want to be health-wise (and life-wise) is simple: track the daily habits that will get you there, and make sure you do them every day. This is how you bypass willpower and discipline (although it might require a bit at the start), how you bypass the stress of goal setting and achievement, and ironically, you get to your goal much faster. Your goal is only whether or not you did 7/7 habits you said you would that week. If you said you'd eat dinner at home each day as a habit, did you do it? If not, what was your adherence rate? 1/7? 3/7? 7/7?

That's the fastest path to getting to where you want to be. Like I said, this is going fly in the face of all the advice you typically get. Set a goal, and feverishly pursue the goal no matter what, right? If you want to actually enjoy your life, and not kill yourself in the process, this is the way to get there stress-free. New goal setting locks you into the present, dispels anxiety, and removes the self hatred and frustration that comes with rigidly viewing goals as black or white.

Chapter Recap: 100 Days of No Goals

☐ **Don't track your goals and the progress bar. Track your habits and your day.** Contrary to most of the advice we get, focusing on goals that are far away usually lead to frustration, depression, and the desire to quit. Fight the desire to thing "I'm XYZ percent towards my goal." Instead, just track whether or not you did the habits today, and this week, that you said you would. Have the goal to know what you want – but forget it, and focus on the daily habits process instead.

☐ **Don't look at the event – the end point – just look at your master the day ritual – the process.** Imagine every day looking at that piece of paper that says, "Lose thirty pounds" and realizing that you're only making .00001% progress each day? Anything you try seems negligible, pointless, and fruitless. That's the problem with most goals, and those are even *realistic* ones – imagine the person that has to lose 100+ pounds? Rather, simply focus on the day-to-day and making each day as perfect as possible. The irony is that when we focus on making smart choices today, without worrying about the progress bar, we get to the end goal much faster – all without guilt and frustration.

The Road to Success

"Success is something you attract by the person you become."

JIM ROHN

Ahh, the road ahead. The road to success. Unfortunately, it's not often *the road to success*. It's not a straight road, anyway. The road to success is usually about as straight as someone drawing a line while having a seizure with a crayon in his hand. I just want to bring up one thing though, so you can prepare for it: You will fail. And guess what? It's okay. We all do. It's not a permanent failure, but sometimes it can feel like it. Sometimes it feels substantial enough that we wonder if it's even worth continuing down the road we're on.

Way back in the chapter on perfectionism and beating yourself up, we talked about how *the process of success creates who we are*. Remember that it's a *process*, not an event. We rarely wake up one day and go "Whoa, I look awesome!" It's a slow curve. Don't forget about wedding day syndrome. One day you wake up and your hip hurts a bit less. The next week you wake up and realize you don't quite feel as mentally foggy. A few months in, you go for a walk and your knees don't hurt anymore. And then over months and years gradually major symptoms turn into minor ones, and then they vaporize into the air. Tiny habits, done daily.

***

Some years ago, my mom decided to take a video camera and start interviewing the elders in our family. We started with her parents who currently live in Las Vegas, and it was my grandma's turn to talk about her life. At one point in the interview she talked about how much she loved and respected her husband, and how he was a major purpose and reason for her being alive. She said one thing in particular that struck me as interesting, when she mentioned hard work, and she said: "He was the hardest working person in his company. If something was wrong with the machinery, he was *the kind of guy that would drive out to the field and fix it himself.*"

Now, my grandpa had anything but an easy life. As an immigrant from Poland who was a child during the great depression in the U.S., he hated talking about his past (and he wouldn't talk about it even if prompted to). His mother was constantly sick and in bed, and his father would bring him to the bar to dance on the counter for money. When I asked what the best advice was that his parents gave him he said, "They didn't give me advice" and quickly changed the subject. He went dumpster diving to feed himself some scraps and snacks, and he couldn't finish a sentence about his childhood without tearing up (hence why he never talked about it).

Flash forward some decades and he had successfully built a massive company – truly from rags to riches, all the while dealing with his own demons. But that one sentence in particular jumped out at me some years later. While reading a book sometime later I stumbled across a Jim Rohn quote that said, "Success is something you attract *by the person you become.*" I thought about that for a minute. I attract success by the person I become? When I went back to that conversation with my grandparents, it made sense. There's a big life lesson here for all of us (especially for our health). My grandpa was *the kind of guy* willing to drive out to the fields and fix his machinery so that his business would run and his team would be happy.

In a world where most of the people running the company would never do that, he was *the kind of guy* that would. Here's the thing: before we take our health to the next level, *we have to take ourselves to the next level*. And that doesn't mean working twice as hard, pushing twice as hard, or exerting twice as much discipline or effort. Not at all. All it means is that we need to cultivate the skills, mindset, resilience, thoughts, beliefs and tools of our next level self.

Let me repeat that. We can't get to the next level of "health" that we want (or life for that matter), until we become the next level version of ourselves. Maybe that's as simple as getting up thirty minutes earlier to meditate. Or maybe that means taking that ten-minute walk before our lunch break at work. Whatever it is, our current self is not getting us to where we want to be. Something has to be upgraded. It's funny, when we look at a success story of something who got crazy fit and healthy after a lifetime of poor health, it can be really temping to think, "Eh, I don't really connect with that story. That person is so far away from where I am... I'm just not that kind of person who can exercise two hours a day. They must be special and have iron discipline." That one phrase is the killer: "I'm just not that kind of person..." I'm not saying we have to spend two hours a day in a gym. But we do need to become the kind of person to achieve whatever levels of health and success we want.

So if the current version of you wakes up late, grabs food to go, stresses out and loses your mind, rushes around all day, and plops down in front of the couch after work – something needs upgrading to get to the next level. As you go through your daily life ask yourself: What would the successful and healthy version of myself do? I've found that it's really interesting how well it works.

- **Current me**: Wake up a half hour before work.
- **Successful me**: Wake up an hour earlier to do the million-dollar *Master the Day* ritual.
- **Current me**: Complain that my spouse always wants me to do the dishes.
- **Successful me**: Do the dishes.
- **Current me**: Know I should start doing yoga because I'm stiff at my desk all day.

- **Successful me**: Sign up for the dang class.

You attract success by *the person you become*. Anytime you're faced with a difficult choice, think about what the "successful" version of yourself would do – this has worked wonders in my own life. What daily habits does the *next level you* cultivate?

What Really Sets Apart Successful "Maintainers" From "Relapsers"

A study done in the American Journal of Clinical Nutrition took 108 women in three different categories:

- Women who maintained their weight loss after formerly being obese
- Women who had always maintained the same, non-obese weight
- Obese women who lost weight but regained it all back

Here were the differences between the successful maintainers (who maintained their new weight), compared to the "relapsers" (who regained the weight back).

1. **Confronted problems directly**: Relapsers (10%), Maintainers (95%)
2. **Used social support**: Relapsers (38%), Maintainers (80%)
3. **Were conscious of behavior** (e.g. eating emotionally)
    1. Relapsers: 70% ate unconsciously in response to emotions
    2. Maintainers: Only 20% ate unconsciously in response to something
4. Relapsers also didn't have many personal strategies for dealing with their own unique situations. Maintainers did.
5. Exercised: Relapsers (34%), Maintainers (90%)[16]

Here's what I find interesting here. Remember *The Key* that is the core theme of this book? Remember the success strategy that I observed in dozens of these 100+ pound weight loss case studies? The only two things you need to succeed are this: understand *The Narrative* (your psychology) and *Little Daily Habits* – and success is inevitable.

Look at two of those markers of success. *Confronted problems directly. Were conscious of behavior.* What I find really interesting is that these are psychological tools! These have nothing to do with eating less and moving more. "Confronted problems directly" meant that these people told the truth. "Something is wrong with my life, and I need to change. What do I need to do differently?" That's it. Okay, I'm gaining weight and feel like crap. What needs to happen? The other group (the relapsers) either went into denial, ignored it, continued to eat emotionally, or did what most of us do: nothing. Psychology. The mind. *The Narrative.* See how powerful it is?

Look at another big one: ate unconsciously in response to emotions. For many of us, cravings are usually the single biggest nutritional issue we deal with as we try to get healthier. There are many nutritional reasons for cravings in a large percentage of people, but in an equally large chunk of people, it's purely emotional. Sitting at our desk around three pm working on a boring work project and we go upstairs or across the street for a cookie or soda? Trigger: Boredom. Have a fight with our spouse or partner, or have a really depressing boring weekend home alone, and have some ice cream? Triggers: Stress and sadness. This is just another reminder that our own mind is the biggest battle when it comes to succeeding at looking and feeling incredible every day.

Everyone wants to sell you some pill or plan – and that's fine -- but nothing will work unless *we change who we are.*

***

What should we do when we get de-railed? Look, it's human. At some point, we're going to be doing great, staying focused, cultivating all these tiny habits that make us successful, healthy and happy… and then *something* will come up. That something is called life. Usually "life" manifests as a Friday night or a holiday. The week went great, you're motivated, inspired, ready to roll, and then it's John's birthday. It's going to be at that restaurant downtown, where everyone is going to be drinking, eating steaks, getting molten lava chocolate cake after their meal, and then downing another few glasses of wine or beer.

You stay focused at the start, but eventually the "oh, *live a little*" ridiculous peer pressure caves us. "Eh, it's just this once," we say. But after the meal – horribly bloated and ready to roll out the restaurant door – the guilt sets in. And the next day is even worse. "Did I just ruin all my hard work? Is it worth even getting back on track today?" This point is where a lot of people quit. It's a small loss, but it feels catastrophic – like your winning streak was just shattered by the opposing team. Sometimes life manifests as getting laid off, having a mid life crisis, watching your relationship crumble and your kids struggle, or some other health or spiritual meltdown that forces you to slow down.

What should you do? Do we wait a while and then begin again? Do we look for a new diet, program or guru? Do we just push harder, and muscle our way to the goal? Whether or not you decide to have cheat days is up to you, but remember this: Whatever you want is on the other side of a couple thousand tiny daily habits. It doesn't require massive work, massive time, or massive discipline and willpower. It just requires changing our daily choices. Remember this?

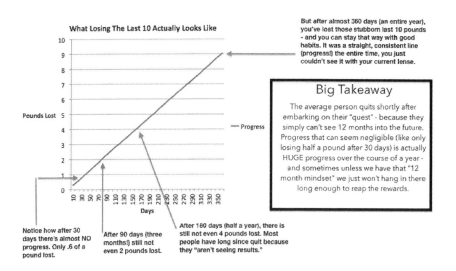

Sometimes when we get derailed the temptation is to go back to the drawing board. "Okay, that diet plan didn't work, maybe I need to find a new, better one customized for me." But that's never the right question. The right question we need to ask ourselves is this: "What was it about my *behavior and habits* that caused me to fail?" Remember: when we understand these habits, we understand that the sooner we take the first step, the sooner we arrive. So if you get sidetracked, just begin again whenever you can.

Rather than seeking out new or different information, sit down for a second and consider what habits led up to that point, and what new habits will get you out of the hole. Remember the daily ritual. If you're keeping up with the daily ritual profiled in the *Master the Day* chapter, you'll naturally want to get back on track. Because you'll be taking five minutes in the evenings, at lunch, or in the mornings to visualize what it is you want, read your little cheat sheet, affirm that you're going to get there, and you'll be inspired to make it happen and *master the day*. This is why this ritual is the foundation of success: it doesn't matter how bad the last day was because each day is a new day, and with your core inspirational/focus routine, you'll re-focus each morning.

Now we're going to hop into one final chapter. At the end of the day, this book is much bigger than just health or weight loss. It's about your life. And being healthy means *freedom*. It means emotional and physical freedom to do everything you want in life and go after those big dreams that have been dormant in your mind and fantasies for decades. It finally gives you permission to wake up from the lifeless zombie haze and begin living the life you really want.

Chapter Recap: The Road to Success

☐   **We will fail and get off track, and it's okay.** Getting derailed is inevitable. For some of us, it happens after the first day or the first week. For some others, we can do incredible for a year, a few years, or even a decade before a major life event messes up the routine and we lose our mojo. Remember: tiny habits, done daily = success. If the dream body comes after 1000 repetitions of a specific set of habits, the sooner we get back to repetition #1, the sooner we arrive at repetition #1,000.

☐   **Relapsers vs. maintainers.** People that successfully maintain their new weight and health habits have five major characteristics based on research:

  ◆   **Confront problems directly** (what's wrong, and how can I fix it?)
  ◆   **Use social support** (should I really be hanging around my old drinking buddies?)
  ◆   **Were conscious of emotional eating behavior** (What's the real reason I'm eating this cookie at 3 pm every day while working on spread sheets?)
  ◆   **Used personal strategies** (Ok, no more binge drinking on Friday, just wine).
  ◆   **Exercised**

☐   **Being healthy will give you your life back.** Health is probably the single most important life habit to cultivate. At the extreme end, no health means death – and you can't do much when you're dead. Everything else is on a spectrum from "great" to "practically dead." Feeling like a million bucks will give you that *oomph* to start doing all the stuff you love in life again.

Beating "Someday Syndrome"

"There are seven days in a week, and someday isn't one of them."

- Unknown

Rewind. It was 2009, and I had just graduated college. I was a fresh recruit, eager with all the ambition and the un-tainted mind of an unrealistic youth. The world was my oyster. Or so I thought. Entering one of the worst job markets on the planet, even though I was a Biology major from a top university, I decided to push the pause button on Medical School. I needed time to figure things out before dropping another decade of my life away and going into multiple six figures of debt.

So I did what any logical person would do. I became a teacher. Teaching is actually pretty cool, especially because I only worked from 8:30 to around three pm. I had the entire summers off, and many of those hours I wasn't necessarily working. Sometimes I just helped students get through a tough part of their lives. A few months into teaching, I was getting antsy. I was twenty-two years old, and with my freshly acquired back pain from sitting at a desk all day, wasn't sure if this was really my passion and purpose in life.

Another experience quickly confirmed that. "Mr. Heyne, please report to the VPs office," the loudspeaker at the school blared. "Wonderful, what goodies are in store for me here?" I thought. Even though I was a teacher, I crept into the Vice Principle's office, to a full committee of about half a dozen district managers, psychiatrists, principles, and more.

"Oh boy."

"Do you know this student?" the *school psychiatrist* asked me as she showed me the picture of a young female. "There have been rumors that you two have been seeing each other outside of school?"

"Uhh, *are you kidding me?*" I asked.

As it turns out, one female student was jealous that *another* female student was "spending time getting tutored by me" (yes, *actually* getting tutored – in school), and thus spread rumors like jealous sixteen-year-old girls do. That made my decision extra easy. I quit at the end of the school year in June, wondered "what next?" in my life, and made yet another logical move: I moved to China. Why China? I had been interested in Kung Fu, meditation, and martial arts since I was a young kid. I was twenty-three now, figured, "This cubicle will always be here for me if I want it to be here, so why not go on an adventure?" So I did the whole kung fu thing: I ate scorpions and some strange foods, I trained three hours a day in the park all in Chinese, learned to speak, read and write Chinese, and had an incredible "bucket list" type year.

But the strangest thing happened. When I returned after checking off a huge item from my bucket list, I spoke with my friends about why they weren't pursuing their big dreams.

"Dude, you're so lucky!" they would tell me.

Ironically, most of them had a bit of money saved, most of them hated their jobs, and most of them were still young, single, and had time. So I asked a close friend, why don't you just go and take a summer off to do some marine biology work in Australia like you always wanted?

"Well, I will *some day.*" And you know what? He sealed his fate right there. For life. As I talked with more and more friends, family and colleagues, this *some day* phrase eerily came up more and more. That's when I decided to do some research.

The Curse of "Some Day"

Someday is a strange phrase. Or rather, it's a phrase we use when we're uncomfortable saying the truth. Think about it, what are some things we say we're going to do "some day?"

- *Some day* I will start getting healthier and lose that beer belly.
- *Some day* I will start my side project, my passion, and see if it takes off.
- *Some day* I will cross that personal project off my bucket list and start!
- *Some day* I will take dance lessons.
- *Some day* I will take my kids, friends, or family out just one on one, and talk about life.
- *Some day* I'll go with my family for a great European vacation in southern France.

One of these days I'll get around to it. It's the ultimate cop out. Behind every one of these, there's an unspoken truth, but we use some day because it's easier to avoid the truth, watch TV, drink or take prescription drugs into oblivion rather than face the facts. The fact is that we're unhappy and we know it, but we're scared of change, we don't think we're good enough, and we're exhausted thinking about how much work it might take for that better life *just* over there.

Life just doesn't feel like the exciting, meaningful adventure it was supposed to be. Here's what "some day" really means underneath. *Some day* I will start getting healthier and lose that beer belly. Here's the unspoken truth: "It seems like a lot of work... I know it's important, but I just struggle to get myself to do it. It sounds tiring, plus I'll have to enter the dating scene again. I don't want to give up all the joys of life either."

Some day I will start my side project, my passion, and see if it takes off. Here's the unspoken truth: "Ehh I don't know, some days after work I'm just tired, plus I have a lot going on with my family and work, and money is tight. I'm afraid of failing, I'm afraid of what people will think, plus what happens if I give it my all and it doesn't work?"

Some day I will cross that personal project off my bucket list and start. Here's the unspoken truth: "I don't really know what I'm passionate about and I don't know the next steps, plus I'd rather watch American Idol and wake up to the same routine 24/7 than do something different and potentially cash in big."

Some day I will take dance lessons. Here's the unspoken truth: "It's just not a priority right now. I work a lot, and I'm pushing my career forward, I've got stuff going on in my relationship and my kids are busy." It's funny - I've always been that kid that asked people why they weren't living the dream. And I mean the exact dream they envisioned. What was holding them back? You'd think it would be specifics like lack of money, time, resources, or know how.

It's not. Overwhelmingly, people just say, "Ehh, it's just…" and then a vague story begins that *they* don't even believe. In other words, lack of urgency. Life may not be great, but it's not bad enough yet that we're shocked into taking action. Sometimes when we finally *do* take action, it's not until later in life when we finally begin to feel the aging process and face our own mortality. Newsflash: This is your life. There is no dress rehearsal - you get one shot. You either are waking up to the life you want, or you aren't. Forget gray area. Don't buy into it. There's a gray area when it comes to your goals, but there isn't a gray area when it comes to your life. Gray area just leads to complacency, stagnation, lack of action and mediocrity. Do we ever wake up and say, "Yeah, I can't *wait* to get up and live a mediocre existence today!" No, of course not.

We all have a terminal illness; it's called *birth*. The thing is, we all understand this intellectually, but we don't really understand this. If we did, we would all live our lives differently. We would take time to kiss our spouse in the morning no matter how grumpy the night before was. We'd slow down in the morning, drink our coffee, and just look out the window and observe the beautiful fall foliage, the snow, the green grass, and the flowers in spring. We'd pause when we sit down to eat. Every sip would be life changing; every bite would be the first bite. And each day, we would stop procrastinating on the things that are so important to us, including our health.

In the end, this book is about your life. Health is such a small part of an incredible life. It's often a barrier to that incredible life though.

Without health, we can't do much. We can't hike mountains in Asia with a bad hip or bum knee. We can't see Machu Picchu if we're out of breath just walking up the stairs to our bedroom. At the end of the day, health is just a vehicle for you to live out your dream, whatever it is. So what's stopping you from getting started?

There are seven days in a week, and some day isn't one of them.

The Gift

"Be careful of your thoughts, for your thoughts become your words.
Be careful of your words, for your words become your actions. Be
careful of your actions, for your actions become your habits. Be
careful of your habits, for your habits become your character. Be
careful of your character, for your character becomes your destiny."

- CHINESE PROVERB

You've been given a priceless gift. That gift is the gift of *choice*. And each moment you have the power to transform your health, happiness, and your life. Each moment you can dramatically change the trajectory of your life. It's *always* in your power. It doesn't matter if we're rich or poor, young or old, male or female, sick or healthy, motivated or unmotivated. We all have the gift. Fill your mind daily with your *why*, with the vision of the future you want.

Remember the two keys: the keys we all have for looking and feeling amazing. The two keys are our inner psychology, the thoughts in our mind and the story we tell ourselves (*The Narrative*), and the daily habits and choices that either pull us to where we want to be, or push us further away. Re-write the story in your head. Pick simple habits that you can do each day to just get 1% better – 1% closer to your goal. Anchor in those habits with daily rituals, routines and emotional anchors. And most of all, don't forget: At the end of the day, health is about freedom. The freedom to do what you want, be who you want, and have what you want, without anything holding you back. So what are you waiting for?

Go on and MASTER THE DAY.

Daily Success Habits

9 Daily Success Habits:

1. It's not about eating less and moving more. It's about trying to juggle all the things we call "life" with being healthy.
2. Tiny daily habits are not only the fastest path to looking and feeling amazing – they're also the easiest path. The millions of seemingly inconsequential daily choices we make create our habits, which dictate our future.
3. Pay attention to *The Narrative*. Re-write it if it's overwhelmingly negative.
4. Create a daily ritual, ideally in the morning. This is a very effective way to actually be consistent with the good habits you are trying to cultivate. Trying to do them at any other time of the day usually fails (especially if you have kids).
5. Write your *why* down on paper. Look at it each morning. Visualize how you want to look and feel. You'd be surprised how well this works.
6. Track your daily habits & review them each week.
7. Write down what new habits need to be cultivated *next* week to improve upon last week (and figure out what didn't work well).
8. If you can't find yourself motivated to do anything, just do one minute, and add one minute per day.
9. Become a process-oriented person. Watch out for wedding day syndrome, focus on *mastering today* and making it as perfect as possible. Just do your best.

The One Page "What to Eat" Guide

Really important here: Don't worry about *when* you eat, or even *how much*. Trust the process (that has worked for hundreds of others), focus on *real food*, avoid anything processed, and cook your own food at least five days a week if you can swing it.

Six Principles:
1. Have 30g protein with each meal
2. Fill half your plate with vegetables (cooked or raw)
3. Put the remainder (about a fistful) filled with low G.I. carbs
4. Remove all liquid calories – including fruit juice (eat your fruit instead).
5. Absolutely avoid: all white bread, white rice, sugar and pasta.
6. Coffee & wine are ok in moderation, and some chocolate is ok – it's important to enjoy life.

What about carbs and fats?
1. Don't remove carbs or be afraid – just eat low G.I. ones
2. Don't remove fats or be afraid – just let your primary sources be olive oil (cooking and dressings), coconut oil (cooking & shakes), avocados, and the fats naturally found in foods like nuts, seeds, and meat.

One day of the week try "eating for energy." This means mostly (or entirely) vegetables & fruits. Avoid coffee, alcohol, meat and grains on this day. Consider it a reboot day. Raw is not necessary.

If this is confusing, there are more bonus resources on my website here: http://modernhealthmonk.com/book/

Notes

[1] Katz, D.L., and S. Meller. "Can We Say What Diet Is Best for Health?" *Annual Reviews*. Annual Review of Public Health: Prevention Research Center, Yale University School of Public Health, Mar. 2004. Web. <http://www.annualreviews.org/doi/full/10.1146/annurev-publhealth-032013-182351>.

[2] Dansinger, Michael. "Comparison of the Atkins, Ornish, Weight Watchers, and Zone Diets for Weight Loss and Heart Disease Risk Reduction." *The Journal of the American Medical Association*. JAMA, 5 Jan. 2005. Web. <http://jama.jamanetwork.com/article.aspx?articleid=200094>.

[3] Lenoir, Magalie *et al*. "Intense Sweetness Surpasses Cocaine Reward." PLOS One, 1 Aug. 2007. Web. 20 Oct. 2015. <http://journals.plos.org/plosone/article?id=10.1371%2Fjournal.pone.0000698>.

[4] Baldo, Brian *et al*. "Wisconsin Study Links Carbohydrate Overeating to Opiate Reaction." *UW School of Medicine and Public Health*. N.p., 03 Feb. 2011.

[5] Steakley, Lia. "The Science of Willpower." *Scope Blog RSS*. SCOPE: Stanford Medicine, 29 Dec. 2011. Web. 20 Oct. 2015. <http://scopeblog.stanford.edu/2011/12/29/a-conversation-about-the-science-of-willpower/>.

[6] Begley, Sharon. "The Brain: How The Brain Rewires Itself." *Time*. Time, 19 Jan. 2007. Web. 20 Oct. 2015. <http://www.time.com/time/magazine/article/0,9171,1580438,00.html>.

[7] Duhigg, Charles. *The Power of Habit: Why We Do What We Do in Life and Business*. New York: Random House, 2012. Print.

[8] De Zwaan, M. "Eating Related and General Psychopathology in Obese Females with Binge Eating Disorder." *Pubmed*. U.S. National Library of Medicine National Institutes of Health, 15 Jan. 1994. Web. <http://www.ncbi.nlm.nih.gov/pubmed/8124326>.

[9] Urquhart, CS *et al.* "Disordered Eating in Women: Implications for the Obesity Pandemic." *Pubmed.Gov*. U.S. National Library of Medicine: NIH, 2011. Web. 21 Oct. 2015. <http://www.ncbi.nlm.nih.gov/pubmed/21382233>.

[10] Stoeber, J *et al.* "Perfectionism and Coping with Daily Failures: Positive Reframing Helps Achieve Satisfaction at the End of the Day." *National Center for Biotechnology Information*. U.S. National Library of Medicine, Oct. 2011. Web. 21 Oct. 2015. <http://www.ncbi.nlm.nih.gov/pubmed/21424944>.

[11] Wiseman, Richard. *The Luck Factor*. London: Arrow, 2004. Print.

12 Steinberg, Dori M *et al.* "The Efficacy of a Daily Self-weighing Weight Loss Intervention Using Smart Scales and E-mail." *Wiley Online Library*. Journal of Obesity, 2 July 2013. Web. 21 Oct. 2015. <http://onlinelibrary.wiley.com/doi/10.1002/oby.20396/abstract>.

[13] Norcross, J.C., Mrykalo, M.S., & Blagys, M.D. (2002). Auld lang syne: Success predictors, change processes, and self-reported outcomes of New Year's resolvers and nonresolvers. *Journal of Clinical Psychology*, 58(4), 397-405.

[14] When choice is demotivating: Can one desire too much of a good thing?

Iyengar, Sheena S.; Lepper, Mark R. Journal of Personality and Social Psychology, Vol 79(6), Dec 2000, 995-1006. <http://dx.doi.org/10.1037/0022-3514.79.6.995>.

15 Rogak, Lisa. *Haunted Heart: The Life and times of Stephen King*. New York: Thomas Dunne, 2009. Print.

16 Kayman, S., W. Bruvold, and JS Stern. "American Journal of Clinical Nutrition: Maintenance and Relapse after Weight Loss in Women: Behavioral Aspects." *National Center for Biotechnology Information*. U.S. National Library of Medicine, Nov. 1990. Web. 22 Oct. 2015. <http://www.ncbi.nlm.nih.gov/pubmed/2239754>.

89769104R00112

Made in the USA
Lexington, KY
02 June 2018